The Secret of Staying Young

Neil Lyall is a well-known food scientist of international repute.
Among other things, he is the inventor of the method by which
potato crisps are flavoured, the 'meatless sausage' and the 'sweet'
cooking of hams and curing of bacon. Many years ago he became
interested in rejuvenation and has spent fourteen years intermittently
researching the ageing process. More recently, he has developed a
tablet form (Pollen-B) of the material which has been held
responsible for the longevity and 'uncommon vitality' of peoples
living in five regions of the world. The results and the sensational
effects of this development are disclosed in this book.

Robert Chapman is equally well known as a science journalist.
He has published a number of books, including one on atomic
energy, and writes on scientific matters in a popular newspaper.
He is a science writer of wide experience and has investigated and
authenticated Lyall's work.

Neil Lyall and Robert Chapman

The Secret of Staying Young

Pollen-B and how it can
prolong your youth

Pan Original
Pan Books London and Sydney

First published 1976 by Pan Books Ltd,
Cavaye Place, London SW10 9PG
© Neil Lyall and Robert Chapman 1976
ISBN 0 330 24781 6
Printed and bound in Great Britain by
Hunt Barnard Printing Ltd, Aylesbury, Bucks

Contents

Illustrations

Acknowledgements

1a Novosti Press Agency
1b Novosti Press Agency
2 *Sunday Express*
3 Popperphoto
4a Oxford Scientific Films
4b Oxford Scientific Films
5a Wassen Developments Ltd
5b Wassen Developments Ltd
6 Norman Potter
7 Studio Lorenzini, Richmond-upon-Thames
8 Norman Potter

'...pollen is the substance of all life in our world. Each grain contains every important substance necessary to a living organism...there would be no life without pollen...'

Dr Naum P. Joirisch
Far East Institute, Soviet Academy of Science
Vladivostok

1 A modern Methuselah

Methuselah, the Bible tells us, lived 969 years. Did he? It seems more than a little likely that he went to join his maker at a very much earlier age – that the incredible figure of 969 has come down to us through an error in communication or transcription. On the other hand, there are grounds for believing that Methuselah remained alive a very long time, for his life would have been frugal, free of stress and lived in open, unpolluted air.

This is certainly true in the case of a modern Methuselah – a Russian fruit farmer who, when he died in September 1973, was said to be 168. By all accounts Shirali Muslimov had lived an idyllic life, though possibly a boring one by modern Western standards, in the Azerbaydzhan mountain village of Barzavu which he hardly ever left. Muslimov, a contemporary of Pushkin and Balzac, was said to have remained, right up to his last days, tending the apple trees in the orchard he had laid down a century earlier. A Moscow news-agency report issued at the time said he was still taking a long walk in the hills each morning. The report also said that Muslimov had celebrated the seventy-fifth anniversary of his marriage to his third wife, Hutun, aged 107. Muslimov could rightly be called a great family man. He left a total of twenty-three children and numerous grandchildren, great-grandchildren and great-great-grandchildren. The tribe of Muslimovs numbered well over two hundred.

Azerbaydzhan holds a leading place for longevity in the Soviet Union. According to statistical data one in every two hundred people in the area is ninety years of age or more. The Russians put Shirali's extreme age down to a combination of ideal circumstances including a near-perfect climate, clean air, plenty of exercise, a well-balanced diet and a lot of sleep (often in the open air). Shirali did not smoke or drink, they say, and even on his birthdays when he received visits and greetings from far and wide he drank only lemonade to toast his guests.

He had never been seriously ill. Pictures of him in recent years show a lean, vigorous-looking old man with a face as keen as a freshly sharpened axe blade, attired in a kaftan-like garment and long boots. He was often seen on horseback and at one time had a reputation as a horseman.

What we have to consider is how much of the amazing story of Shirali Muslimov is the precise truth and how much deliberate or fortuitous eyewash. Is there for example any documentary evidence that he was 168 years old when he died? Any birth certificate, for example? And what about other villagers still alive and approaching Muslimov's age . . . some of whom may have even exceeded it?

Have the peoples of Azerbaydzhan some survival advantages missing from our own way of life? And while considering this it should not be overlooked that the USSR is not the only country in the world where the phenomenon of extreme old age in good health is to be found. There are also places like Vilcabamba Valley in Ecuador, the neighbouring state of Colombia, and Hunza in Pakistan.

If *you* have reached the age of seventy in good shape you are doing all right. Three score years and ten has long been considered the allotted span. But the average length of life for humanity is increasing all the time. Soon we may have to abandon the old figures for something more realistic – perhaps as high as four score years and five. To achieve such an average, however, a great many people will have to live much longer, to compensate for those who, for one reason or another, die younger.

In an article published by the United Nations Educational, Scientific and Cultural Organization, Professor Dmitri Chebotarev of the Soviet Union's Institute of Gerontology said that there were more than 112 million active men and women over the age of seventy in the world today and this total was increasing all the time.

Just how long people in general could continue to survive if they never had any illnesses is not known but it is thought that 125 years would not be an unrealistic figure. Some predictions push the age limit up as high as 150 and a few medical authorities, notably Dr Lawrence E. Lamb, former professor of Medicine at America's Baylor University, have gone as far as predicting a time (in the not-too-distant future) when, apart from succumbing to the effects of serious diseases, accidents or violence at the hands of others, man need never die at all unless he wishes to do so.

At this moment it is believed there are 250,000 people over a hundred in different parts of the world. A large number, according to Chebotarev, appear to reside in rural areas of the USSR. But vigorous hundred-year-olds are also living in numbers in other countries, some of which have become famous for their lively, high-spirited centenarians.

Of course, there is little to be gained in living to a hundred years or more if you are bedridden or a liability to other people, especially relatives, or if you are chronically sick or in pain. Living into your second century can only be worthwhile if you remain in good health, with undiminished faculties, and can play a useful part in community life. What is desired is not to grow older but to stay younger longer.

So the purpose of this book is to look at the ageing situation as it is today; to account, if possible, for the dramatic turn that ideas of longevity seem to have taken; to test the validity of claims that some people are already living well into their second century; to evaluate predictions that death may ultimately be defeated and to ask ourselves what new problems, even dangers, may lurk along the path to immortality.

It is proposed to release details of a fourteen-year-long research programme leading to the development of a substance that early experiments indicate may play an important part in keeping us all fit and well long past the time when so many, if only subconsciously, begin to feel it is not worth going on.

The questions to be considered are these. Is it simply that the people of these long-living regions enjoy ideal climatic conditions and occupy themselves in ways that enable them to avoid stress? Is it that, consciously or otherwise, they know what is best for them to eat or drink? Or could there be something else – another factor of which even they themselves may be unaware . . . which keeps them going long after their contemporaries in the world at large have given up the ghost?

*

No consideration of ageing and eventual death can really be made without a notion of what we mean by life. So what is life, as far as humanity is concerned?

Basically, it is awareness of one's existence and environment. All land animals, fishes, birds and insects appear to have this awareness to some extent. There is even a dawning belief among researchers that still life, as we think of the vegetation of this planet, is not all that still but that trees and flowers and shrubs all know in some strange fashion that they are alive.

Every living creature is a source of infinite wonder, but none more so than Man, with his reasoning power, his inventiveness and his boundless imagination. The human body is staggeringly complex, so much so indeed that we are only on the threshold of understanding how it works; how it develops from infancy to maturity and on to old age; how it reproduces itself in conformity with an incredibly detailed hereditary pattern.

Not the least remarkable aspect of the living body concerns the bewildering network of nerve pathways, all flashing electric signals every second of time to and fro between the brain and every part of our being, so that the brain is constantly informed, constantly processing the information, constantly acting upon it.

The brain is the most elaborate instrument in all earthly creation. It is made of billions of parts called neurons directly or potentially connected to one another. All the telephone, telegraph, radio and radar apparatus in the world is less intricate than the three pounds or so of 'grey matter' in the human skull. Quite literally, we do not know what we are doing most of the time; the brain does it for us.

Just think of all the detailed adjustments of movement and balance that enable us simply to walk down the street without falling over. Think of a cricketer in the outfield running to catch a ball, calculating its flight path as he positions himself so that the ball falls safely into his cupped hands. Think of what is involved in making the noises we call speech . . . how we can distinguish one sound from another and even determine pretty well the distance and direction from which they come.

Think of our marvellous ability to distinguish fine shades of colour, to solve intricate problems, to recall events going back half a century or more. Think of the way we can learn to play the piano, use a typewriter, drive a car or ride a bicycle without giving conscious thought to the mechanism of the particular skill involved. Yet every tiny action is the result of a nerve signal controlled by the brain; and when we become tired the brain can switch us off for a few hours to give our bodies – and perhaps itself as well – a rest.

Nobody can construct a human brain. Indeed it has been estimated that to build even a crude model would require billions of transistors, an equal number of wires, a warehouse hundreds of times the size of the average living-room and at least a million kilowatts of electrical power. Yet our brains manage on a mere 25 watts, casually carrying out work programmes that would baffle the most elaborate computer in existence.

In our daily lives we take ourselves very much for granted. If we are hungry we eat; if thirsty we drink; if tired we lie down. If we are hot we make for the shade; if cold we seek the means to get warm. If we are bored we look for entertainment; if frightened we run. We rarely question anything about ourselves; hardly ever wonder whether we are looking after ourselves properly, taking risks, damaging our bodies unnecessarily. And much the same applies to growing old. In youth we hardly give it a thought. Then, as the years pile up, we find ourselves gradually accepting what we regard as inevitable. After all, it happens to everybody, doesn't it? You don't hear so well and you may have to resort to a deaf-aid. Your eyes weaken and you need even stronger spectacles. You get breathless quickly. Odd pains occur in the back, the arms and the legs. Every physical effort becomes more taxing. But there's always the television. It's good to sit down and fall asleep in front of the telly.

And the years roll on . . .

2 Seeking an elixir of life

'There's night and day, brother, both sweet things; sun, moon and stars, brother, all sweet things; there's likewise a wind on the heath. Life is very sweet, brother; who would wish to die?' GEORGE BORROW

Men throughout the ages have often felt like the author of *Lavengro*. Probably the earliest primitive savage, scratching his puzzled head in the flowing wilderness of pre-history, thought mournfully of the time when he would grow old and life would be taken from him.

For thousands of years men have sought ways of delaying death, but it was only comparatively recently that the search for magic medicine, an elixir of life, assumed academic status. The idea of increasing longevity was a favourite one with the ancient Egyptians who thought that making themselves sick at regular intervals, and also sweating heavily, would help them remain youthful longer, an idea which has reappeared in Turkish and sauna baths. The elderly would also surround themselves with young people – a practice which is not unknown today – in the hope of bolstering their flagging energies and preserving good looks with the 'effluvia of blooming youth'. But in case it did not work, the Egyptians had another idea. They were the first people to postulate the notion of an after-life that, if lacking the reality of that enjoyed by their physical bodies before death, would not be as bad as total extinction.

In Roman times, the breath of young maidens was thought to have a powerful effect in warding off old age. And no doubt many a rich Roman, whether or not he sincerely believed in the remedy, had his latter years sweetened by close contact with pretty girls employed to treat him. For a long time afterwards, however, it does not appear that much attention was paid to the notion of living to a great age. But in the mid eighteenth century a gentleman calling himself the Count of St Germain gained enormous popularity both in London and on the Continent for his discovery of the 'Tea of Long Life'. But his wild claim that anyone drinking the tea regularly would reach a ripe old age of two thousand years, took a severe knock when the Count himself died at seventy . . . or with 1,930 years still to go! The tea was later found to be a simple mixture of senna, fennel and sandalwood.

Cagliostro, the Italian charlatan, who visited London in 1771, was another bogus Count (real name Joseph Palsamo). He claimed to have discovered a long-life elixir along with an assortment of love philtres and beauty lotions. Cagliostro conned his way all over Europe and was nobly entertained by kings and potentates. But, like Count St Germain, he eventually died, miserably and in disgrace, when he was only fifty-two. Cagliostro's death-defying elixir was nothing more than a commonplace remedy for indigestion. Many quacks and charlatans cashed in on the gullibility of an unprotected public before the modern Medicines Act of the Department of Health and the vast range of current food regulations were formulated to protect consumers from such exploitation.

Yet in more modern times, in 1960 to be precise, astonished newspaper readers in Britain were told of a potion named 'Exultation of Flowers' being sold from a house in Scotland by a retired bank manager and an ex-nurse. The couple were offering two ounce bottles for 14/3d (old currency). They declared that the potion would keep men and women feeling young and looking perfectly fit throughout their lives.

At the same time it was admitted with commendable honesty that the 'Exultation of Flowers' would be analysed by a chemist as nothing more elaborate than water. What the water contained, however, the couple claimed was the 'potencies' of fifty-two different flowers, for they had discovered a way of channelling the electrical impulses given off by flowers and transferring them to water.

It was a secret known only to themselves. The former *Daily Sketch* quoted the ex-nurse as saying: 'The potion increases the vitality of all living things. It removes every type of disease from the body. We have no expensive equipment and we treat the water ourselves, transferring the electrical impulses to bowls of water.'

Not the least important feature of this 'Exultation of Flowers' was that it increased human confidence. The newspaper commented that anyone with the confidence to pay 14/3d for a bottle of water did not need an elixir.

Another substance, which appeared to offer some prospects of restoring lost youth and maintaining it, excited all Paris in the 1950s. It was called 'orthobiotique serum' and was prepared in the famous Pasteur Institute from the prescription of a Russian research doctor named Alexander Bogomoletz. The serum was made by extracting bone marrow from a healthy human being and injecting it into the

19

bloodstream of a horse from which it was later separated again. The action of this serum was thought to stave off the ageing process by preventing the destruction of connective tissues surrounding all human organs. 'Man is as old as his connective tissues,' Bogomoletz was supposed to have remarked.

Some remarkable instances of restored virility were reported by the use of 'orthobiotique serum'. But a leading biologist of the day, Dr Maurice Ernest, put the damper on any enthusiasm for the serum in Britain. After forty-five years' study in gerontology and experiments on thirty thousand patients, he was quoted in the *Sunday Pictorial* as saying: 'How can you put Youth into a medicine bottle for universal distribution when all our bodies are as individually different as our fingerprints? But there is no reason,' he added, 'why we should not all live to a hundred or even two hundred years of age. Youthfulness can be preserved by preventing the organic disorders which cause senile degeneration.'

Possibly the first scientific, certainly the first surgical method of rejuvenation attempted was that known as the monkey gland treatment. Its impact on the medical world, if not the world in general, was explosive and even now, some sixty years later, faint echoes of that impact continue to reverberate from time to time. Ask anyone of middle-age what he knows of monkey gland treatment and you will at least get the reply that 'it had something to do with making people young again, didn't it?' The name Voronoff might even be recalled.

Serge Voronoff was a Russian working in France who had the idea that ageing was basically associated with the decline in sexual virility . . . a notion that came to him when he was employed as a harem doctor in Egypt and was struck by the fact that the eunuchs tended to die around the age of sixty, looking much older than their years. Voronoff reasoned that if an elderly man's testicular function could be boosted by transplant surgery, that man would have youthful vigour and vitality restored to him.

To begin with, Voronoff supposed that such operations might be carried out with help from human volunteers in return for attractive cash rewards which wealthy patients would be only too pleased to pay. But it did not work. Not surprisingly, perhaps, volunteers were hard to find. In fact, no acceptable volunteers were found at all.

Undaunted, Voronoff turned his attention to chimpanzees – who were not in a position to argue, and for years he continued to transplant these 'monkey glands' (how else could one express it in those days?) into the scrota of rich elderly patients who were 'past it' but could afford to go back for another try. Alas; any improvements were only temporary, and in some cases, perhaps imaginary.

Though perhaps a trifle dogmatic in his approach, Voronoff was not demonstrably a fraud. One cannot, however, take such a tolerant view of Voronoff's American counterpart, Dr John Brinkley of Kansas who, in the same heyday of sexual transplants (just after the First World War) had his licence to practise medicine taken from him. Instead of using chimpanzees, Brinkley used goats (largely because of their reputation for tireless mating) and is reported to have carried out sixteen thousand transplants before it was realized that he was blatantly cashing in on the credulity of patients.

Early attempts to rejuvenate the elderly were always carried out at enormous fees and even medical men like Brinkley made fortunes out of the gullibility of wealthy patients. Explanations were rarely given and few patients admitted having such treatments. Consequently no recommendations or testimonials were available. The operations were carried out in an atmosphere of some secrecy although wild claims were often made for their success. In fact, no 'rejuvenation treatment', from St Germain down to Voronoff, was subject to legal or medical authority and all invariably failed.

Today, medical and advertising standards committees, as well as medical consultants to large newspaper groups, technical journals and retail chemists' groups, carefully check products available to the public and thus safeguard us from being misled or overcharged. Public analysts, too, examine every product and its ingredients and there are even consumer organizations to give further protection.

Several ideas from the past can, of course, be modified for use today and, as already noted, it is possible that the heavy sweating of ancient Egyptian culture has reappeared in Turkish and sauna baths. Sweating can remove toxins from the body through the pores of the skin.

The Count of St Germain and Voronoff at least played their part in arousing interest in prolonging vigorous and active life and, to some extent, supporting the notion that death is due to disease or accident rather than sheer old age.

3 Cell therapy and GH3

It is difficult, and becoming more so, for anyone nowadays to hoodwink the public with a bogus preparation for prolonging active life and vitality. We are all that much more enlightened than our forebears – perhaps cynical would not be an inappropriate word to use. Anyway, we rightly suspect the medicament which evidence suggests was concocted in a back garden shed rather than being properly developed by qualified scientists working under sterile laboratory conditions. We know, too, that should the preparation contain a drug it must come to us with the approval of the government's Medicines Committee which now replaces the former Safety of Drugs Committee, and only after testing and examination to ensure not only safety but, to some extent, effectiveness.

It can be assumed therefore that substances (no longer to be accurately described as 'elixirs') mentioned from here on are all genuine in the sense that they have serious scientific backing even if it cannot be said that they have added much to the sum of human knowledge about ageing, still less have had a lasting effect upon the human body.

In 1958 representatives of an organization called Institut d'Etudes des Biocatalyseurs came to Britain to extol the merits of a substance known as royal jelly. They proclaimed that it opened up new horizons enabling man to re-establish his 'biological balance' and face his later years with serenity and optimism.

If you are a bee-keeper you will know immediately what is meant by royal jelly. It is a clear, viscous liquor secreted from the salivary glands of the worker bee, and contains soluble ingredients of pollen as well as traces of nectar. Worker bees regurgitate royal jelly to feed the queen (hence its name, of course). They also feed the very young bee larvae on this material. Royal jelly is a dilute solution of these pollen ingredients, but it is a readily digestible liquid food. The extreme care taken by the workers of their queen enables her to live an average life of between three and five years whereas the workers literally work themselves to death in about forty to fifty days. Royal jelly, while sufficiently nourishing for the queen, contains about 75 per cent of water. According to a *Times* medical report, the longer life of the queen may be partly due to the fact that, although she lays a prodigious quantity of eggs, about three thousand every day, she uses only a fraction of the energy of the worker bees. Said the *Times*: 'Clinical reports on the value of royal jelly, coming mainly from the Continent, are so confusing as to be meaningless. Apart from anything else, there is no method of standardizing the jelly for human use. The dosage is so small that even the known ingredients could have little effect, if any.'

While a multiplicity of claims was formerly made for it, it seems far more likely that the value of royal jelly was largely psychological, due to the glamour and novelty of the treatment.

*

The human body, in common with the animal body, the

24

insect body, the body of every living thing on earth including the denizens of the vegetable kingdom, is made up of billions of microscopic particles called cells, each consisting of a nucleus surrounded by its own portion of less dense tissue. Growth, whether of flesh or bone, teeth or hair or fingernails, is caused by the multiplication of these cells in a process known as cell-division, when one cell splits to form two identical cells. But some cells die. Indeed, it is estimated that throughout the human body as a whole, millions of cells die every week. Fortunately, the dead ones are immediately replaced by the constant division of neighbouring cells.

In the case of disease and ageing (which some specialists believe is itself a form of disease) the rate of production of cells falls below the rate of dying cells, causing a critical imbalance in certain areas of the system. What follows is something anyone can observe for himself – loss of elasticity of the skin, for example, stiffening of the joints, thinning or whitening of the hair. More significantly, however, there is a decrease in brain cells, the reduction of lung capacity, a falling-off of reflex reactions, lowering of body temperature and the degeneration of reproductive organs – all symptoms of ageing and partial death of the organism.

So it is plainly important to our wellbeing that we keep our cell production working. But suppose we cannot do it for ourselves? Is there any way in which we can get help? The answer many experienced people will give you is an emphatic 'Yes'. For more than forty years, the practice of what is termed 'cell therapy' has been going on in different countries.

It all started in 1931, when Professor Paul Niehans was called upon to help a young surgeon with an emergency operation. The surgeon was operating on a woman patient for goitre, a condition which affects the thyroid gland of the neck. The surgeon's hand had slipped and damaged the tiny parathyroid glands which are situated near the thyroid gland. The result was to bring about a condition known as tetany which is normally fatal. The patient automatically developed the cramp-like muscular spasm of tetany and the only possible action to save the woman was to graft new parathyroid glands.

Professor Niehans arrived at the clinic after collecting the parathyroid glands of a young steer calf from a nearby abattoir but realized that the patient's condition was too critical to survive a grafting operation. Instead, he cut up the steer glands into very minute portions, made them into a solution and injected this into the patient's breast muscle. Almost immediately the tetany disappeared and the patient recovered. She continued to improve and eventually lived another thirty years. This was the beginning of cell therapy as it is known today.

Nowadays the cells used are obtained from the foetuses of sheep about a month from the date of expected birth. Cells may be obtained, for example, from the heart, liver or other organs. The practice then is to determine the type of cells in which a particular patient appears to be deficient, and inject a solution of appropriate or matching sheep cells to boost areas in need of them. The injected cells reach their target by a sort of natural 'magnetic' attraction. For example, should a patient have a liver condition, then fresh liver cells are used to stimulate the patient's own liver cells. In other words, the injected cells travel only to the corresponding organ or gland for which they have a specific affinity.

An information pamphlet issued in London by the Cell Therapy Centre tells us: 'After treatment, patients report that they feel much more relaxed and that they are better able to cope with their stress-filled lives. They sleep better and feel less anxious and worried because their nervous system has been toned up.'

Organically, too, the patient's system improves. Digestive disturbances react well to this treatment and so do conditions involving the heart and the arteries. The liver and kidneys are frequently treated by this method. Indeed it is possible to treat any part of the human body. Impotence and frigidity are among the most common cases treated by the Centre. Others include menopause and menstruation difficulties. Overweight and lack of skin texture and muscle tone are also conditions which react favourably to this treatment.

Cell therapy can achieve many dramatic improvements and it appears to be one of the more effective modern devices. Most of all, it gives the body a better resistance to disease, and gives the patient a much fuller and often longer life without the unpleasantness so often accepted as inevitable with ageing and the ageing process.

The practitioners of cell therapy claim that many international figures have sought their treatment. The list of the illustrious is said to have included Sir Winston Churchill, Charles de Gaulle, the Duke and Duchess of Windsor, Konrad Adenauer, Somerset Maugham, General Eisenhower, the Japanese Imperial Family, King Ibn Saud, Marlene Dietrich, Charlie Chaplin, the Duke of Sutherland, Gloria Swanson, Gaylord Hauser and Pope Pius XII who is reported to have publicly blessed the treatment.

Unlike some of his predecessors, Paul Niehans never

claimed that his treatment could keep anyone alive indefinitely but only that the injection of young cells into an old body could rejuvenate it in the sense that a better life was possible throughout the natural span, provided former bad habits were abandoned.

*

The aircraft bringing Professor Ana Aslan from Bucharest, Romania, landed at London airport on 18 November 1959. A crowd of journalists and cameramen surged forward to greet her and were astonished at what they saw. Professor Aslan was said to be in her sixties but, with her elegant bearing and smooth skin, the light in her eyes and the sheen in her hair, she hardly looked forty. It no longer seemed impossible that she had discovered the secret of youth; nor was it difficult to believe the many stories that had preceded her, of old people shuffling into her clinic in the Romanian capital and lightly stepping out again as if they had shed twenty years or more.

Professor Aslan, as the world soon learned, had 'discovered' a white, soluble crystalline substance known as procaine hydrochloride (widely used in dentistry as a local anaesthetic) and re-named it Gerovital H3, later to be known as GH3. Injections of a solution of this material, it was claimed, could improve the impaired hearing of premature senility, loosen old arthritic joints, reverse hardening of the arteries, make wrinkled skin smooth again, put colour back into hair gone snowy with age and impart new vigour to the elderly.

Everyone in Bucharest at the time had heard of the classic case of the country's ageing star, actress Lucea Blandra. When, at the age of seventy-eight it was said, Lucea had first sought treatment at the Institute of Geriatrics she was feeble and confused and had the greatest difficulty remembering her lines. Now she was eighty-five, playing the leading role in a play by George Bernard Shaw and directing two other plays at the same time. No wonder people said she had become a new woman. And there were said to be similar cases, some of even more illustrious patients. Ho Chi-Minh was said to have benefited. Kwame Nkruma, too, and one of President Sukarno's wives.

GH3 was not the result of planned research. Professor Aslan had been using a solution of procaine hydrochloride in her capacity as a doctor to treat patients suffering from rheumatism. She then noticed that not only was the rheumatism relieved but skin troubles cleared up and people seemed to become more active in mind and body. She experimented with animals and finally came to the conclusion that she had found a remarkable new use for an old substance. Professor Ana Aslan had gratifying support from Dr Hewlett Johnson, the Red Dean of Canterbury, who visited her clinic in Bucharest when he was over eighty. The Dean said afterwards, 'I had a course of her treatment, which has had an extraordinarily happy effect on me – restoring powers that I had lost. It made me feel and act as if several years had been taken off my age.'

Later it was reported that Professor Aslan had been to Moscow and China to treat top Communists and by now her fame was spreading through the West as well. A British newspaper headline proclaimed: REDS FIND CURE FOR OLD AGE. But it was a year before Ana Aslan was invited to tell the story of her discovery in Britain. She arrived carrying a bunch of red carnations and a bag containing one hundred ampoules of GH3, to receive the full celebrity treatment, including

29

dinner at the House of Commons and lunch at the House of Lords. She was interviewed over and over again. The telephone in her Kensington hotel room hardly ever stopped ringing.

But what Ana Aslan had come for was to confer with British doctors. And the time came when she faced two hundred of them in London's Apothecaries' Hall. She told them with modesty and charm of her many successes with GH3, and the doctors listened with genuine interest and put questions to which she always had an answer. At the end there was warm-hearted applause and a vote of thanks to the visitor. But, as Cedric Carne reported in the *Sunday Express*, the next issue of the *British Medical Journal* was distinctly unflattering to her. It said:

'A study of the clinical reports makes sad reading for the clinician trained in modern scientific method. There is an almost complete absence of controls and blind trials were never used. At the Apothecaries' Hall . . . Professor Aslan created a favourable impression as a woman gifted with humour, charm, enthusiasm and boundless therapeutic optimism. The word "statistical" was heard frequently but no worthwhile statistics were shown. The audience heard little but a series of medical anecdotes.'

Those who carried out extensive clinical tests with GH3 after Professor Aslan's return to her own country reported that they had been 'a complete flop'. Sixty-four patients, it was said, had been treated for twelve months but the doctors in charge found that the injections were of no value. The last word on the subject at the time was spoken by Dr Alex Comfort, a leading British researcher into the causes of ageing. 'Dr Aslan,' he said, 'is a completely sincere woman and her substance does lead to some curious results. But, as yet, there is no scientific evidence that it is of real use in old age.'

But, as usual, that was not the end of the matter. In September 1974 the *Sunday Express* published a story under the headline:

BEDFORD IS BEING REJEVENATED IN A BUCHAREST CLINIC

'The Duke of Bedford, a sprightly fifty-six, is having private medical care behind the Iron Curtain. He and his wife Nicole are at the Romanian State Institute of Geriatrics in Bucharest – otherwise known as the Aslan Clinic for Rejuvenation.

'This clinic, which is quietly favoured by several wealthy English people – the Begum Aga Khan is also there at the moment – is run by Professor Ana Aslan, seventy-six. Professor Aslan has said that, with the help of her miracle drug GH3, a person might possibly be able to live to 130 years.'

The Duke of Bedford was quoted as saying, 'No, I don't want to live for ever but I do hope I can get rid of the aches and pains which you get when you grow old.'

It is the mild analgesic effect of procaine hydrochloride that appears to be its main appeal but British pharmaceutical manufacturers have described Ana Aslan's therapy as 'indecisive'. Similar relief from aches and pains could, in fact, have been achieved with paracetamol or some other pain-killing drug. A German version of procaine therapy known as KH3 and involving the use of tablets to be taken orally is also considered 'indecisive' in its effects.

*

There are, of course, a number of preparations on the market which, it is claimed, 'put new life' into people lacking energy from middle-age onwards. Most of these buck-you-up remedies probably do have some beneficial effect, especially to those who have faith in them, but all should be regarded with suspicion.

Some, it is claimed, will restore sexual potency in ageing men, keep hair from falling out, overcome lassitude and, if not actually adding years to the life-span, at least make the latter years more vigorous and interesting. But the operative word is 'claimed', for there exists no evidence that would satisfy unbiased scientific inquiry.

One preparation gaining popularity in the Western world nowadays contains an ancient Chinese remedy known for hundreds of years. The Chinese call it 'ginseng', meaning 'man-plant', because the principal ingredient comes from a common plant with roots that are said to resemble the figure of a man. But unlike man, who is a gregarious creature, the ginseng plant seems rather shy and tends to grow best in deeply shaded woodlands and hillsides, particularly in Manchuria.

The modern Chinese are said to use the root to make a health-giving kind of 'tea' which they brew in silver kettles; others simply chew the root raw and swallow its juices. When Marco Polo travelled through China in 1274, he reported finding ginseng in general use as a panacea for all diseases. But hardly anything appears to have been done over the years to discover whether the ginseng root contains anything of real value to humanity.

Neil Lyall, who has examined nearly every known preparation said to have revitalizing properties, assigns ginseng to the long list of 'folk medicines' which have come briefly to prominence over the past thousand years. The list includes wheat-germ oil, oil of garlic and even pantocrine – an extract from the antlers of the Siberian spotted deer!

They may contain trace elements of beneficial materials, he says, but certainly not enough to be of lasting value. As ginseng consists mostly of insoluble fibres, the amount of assimilable nourishment must be very small indeed.

4 Police sweat it out

Mankind, we believe, was cradled in the sea.

We gradually grew up from primitive organisms that crawled uneasily out of the shallows, millions of years ago, to make a new life on the land. In a sense we still have the sea with us in the form of the blood and water streams that clean and nourish our body cells just as the warm oceans of the world once cleansed and nourished the cells of primeval life.

The sea, in fact, may have played a more important part in the evolution of Man than is generally realized, not only creating and sending him forth but later reshaping and re-educating him for the long and hazardous journey to the door of civilization. This, at any rate, is the view of the eminent marine biologist, Sir Alister Hardy.

Sir Alister's theory is that almost a million years ago some of our remote and hairy ancestors, hardly distinguishable from true apes, went back into the shallow seas to hunt for food, making their homes along the shore. Slowly, over the ages, they learned to swim. This caused them to develop longer legs and more sensitive fingers for feeling along the sea-bed and opening shell-fish; meanwhile they also lost the hair from their bodies but retained it on their heads to protect them from the sun.

Supported by the water, the theory goes, they learned to stand erect. They picked up stones from the beaches to use as rudimentary tools, particularly to crack the shells of crabs and other fish. From then onwards it was only a short step to discovering that certain stones could be chipped into shape to make primitive knives and sharp-pointed tips for spears and arrows.

So, when the sea-ape came away from the seas about five hundred thousand years later, he was already almost a man with the intelligence and agility to dominate other land creatures. He could now proceed to conquer the continents – running and hunting the animals of the plains.

Be that as it may, the fact remains that we are still fundamentally water creatures. At least 70 per cent of the weight of the human body consists of water, carrying in solution all the nutrients that the cells need for a healthy and vigorous life.

The simplest form of life is the single-cell amoeba. It lives in water from which it absorbs food and oxygen. And into the water it excretes waste products and carbon dioxide gas after it has converted its food into energy. The amoeba uses its skin for ingesting food, breathing and rejecting waste. If it cannot get the right foods and oxygen it dies. And it also dies if the water surrounding it becomes contaminated by impurities, including its own waste products.

Since our bodies are made up of billions of microscopic cells, each resembling the amoeba, it follows that it is vitally important that the warm salty water around them is never allowed to become impure and stagnant. In fact, the major excretory organs of the body such as the kidneys, liver and lungs are largely occupied in eliminating waste products such as urine, bile and carbon dioxide taken from the cell water.

So the ancient Egyptians were not wrong in thinking that hot baths and sweating were good for us, removing toxins from the body through the pores of the skin. Even when we are not doing heavy work, there is a continuous evaporation of sweat from the pores or sweat glands on the surface of the skin. Indeed, a man whose job involves sitting at his desk in an air-conditioned office may lose a pint of body water in the course of twenty-four hours, providing himself with a splendid excuse for calling in at the pub on his way home.

The human skin is the largest organ of the body and is a kind of lattice that opens and closes to help us maintain a constant body temperature of 37 degrees Centigrade (98.6 degrees Fahrenheit). If two-thirds of the body's surface were tarred over, thus stopping up the pores, a man would die, not only through over-heating but because he could not rid himself of harmful substances which normally pass out through the pores. Sweating, as everyone knows, invariably brings relief in illness, especially in cases like pneumonia and malaria, where high temperatures are involved.

The cold sweat produced by shock, coronary thrombosis and vascular disease when death is near represents the last attempt of the body to rid itself of poisons and carbon dioxide. This was noted by Dr Nathaniel Hodges as long ago as the Plague of London in 1665. The doctor recorded that brackish and profuse sweats gave a good prognosis but that cold and watery sweats were soon followed by death. Both Dr Hodges and a colleague, Dr Thomson of Houndsditch, survived the plague. The latter made a point of sweating every day by getting into a bed warmed with hot bricks and taking a bottle of sack and an ounce of dark treacle.

There is evidence that deliberate sweating as a means of

37

maintaining health and vitality and prolonging life has been practised since the beginning of civilization long before anyone knew precisely what effect it had. People just felt better. Thus, for example, the Romans, during their occupation of Britain two thousand years ago, were always popping in and out of specially heated rooms at their communal bath houses. An example of these still exists at Chedworth Roman Villa in Gloucestershire. Today we have the saunas and Turkish baths where men and women can go to have the toxic effects of over-eating and drinking sweated out of their systems. But it has been only during the past two decades that the basic therapeutic value of exercising the sweat glands has been studied in detail.

When the City of London's £2½ million Police Headquarters in Wood Street was opened by the Lord Mayor in 1966, it was learned that a special health unit designed to keep men in the pink of condition had been built in the basement. This unit, it was reported, would not only help them to avoid winter coughs and colds but would prevent heart attacks – a splendid contribution to longevity – and generally counteract the physical process of ageing. Somehow, it did not get a great deal of publicity but this unit, still in use, was the first of its kind in the world – the outcome of more than twelve years' research by a pioneer physician, Dr Eric St John Lyburn of Tunbridge Wells, Kent.

Basically, this unit is a 'Turkish bath', but it has refinements resulting from thousands of experiments aimed at understanding the complex mechanisms of the human body – in particular the action of the sweat glands. Dr Lyburn's researches are based on the conviction that good health is dependent upon the speedy removal of poisons that accumulate in the ordinary course of living.

In youth, this removal is efficiently carried out by the kidneys, he explains, but in later years, the kidneys begin to fail and find it increasingly difficult to do their work. As a result arthritis, rheumatism and similar diseases begin to afflict us. Even people who feel quite well may be suffering from the onset of slowly developing diseases of this kind. But there is a way of checking them and, in so doing, keeping old age at bay.

Under carefully controlled conditions in which the head is cooled in a stream of ice-cold air the body can be superheated, causing not just ordinary sweating but a torrent of perspiration that could not be achieved in the normal way by violent exercise even in a Turkish or sauna bath.

Men taking the Lyburn treatment in the City unit strip off and sit in wooden cubicles in a white-tiled steam room. The temperature of the room rises from 37 to 49 degrees Centigrade (100 to 120 degrees Fahrenheit). But, though perspiring profusely, they feel no discomfort. Their heads are enclosed in special cowls enabling them to breathe cold air from a separately piped supply. Meanwhile the constant high temperature below their necks ensures that perspiration cannot evaporate and cool their bodies in the normal way. Instead, their sweat glands are kept constantly active releasing used cell water and its impurities. To compensate for the rapid loss of water, cold drinks are provided.

Dr Lyburn's experiments have shown that regular half-hour periods of this treatment leave a man (or woman) feeling fresh and invigorated, and he says, 'Head-cooling not only makes the treatment pleasurable but fools the nervous system into releasing control of the sweat glands, which then act rather like auxiliary kidneys helping to expel poisonous wastes and germs. At the same time oxygen is able to reach the bloodstream through the opened-up skin tissue and assist the lungs.'

The process of ageing, he believes, starts with the failure of the kidneys and liver to do their work adequately. Consequently, if some of the work-load is taken off them from time to time the business of growing old is significantly retarded.

Most of Dr Lyburn's research has been carried out at the Tunbridge Wells spa where he also treats patients, not only from his own locality but from all over the country and all over the world. Tunbridge Wells once ranked with Bath, Cheltenham and Leamington as a place where wealthy invalids went to 'take the waters' – usually for gout. What, if anything, made the difference was that the spa waters had an exceptionally high mineral content, mainly of iron salts. Of course, if combined with a diet rich in vitamins, enzymes and amino acids this could be very beneficial.

The Tunbridge Wells spring was discovered by Lord North in the time of James I. History records that about 1735 Beau Nash left Bath to become Master of Ceremonies at Tunbridge Wells – which led to a well-ordered round of social gatherings and activities often favoured by royalty.

But, in the course of time, even the rich began to realize that the spa water alone was doing limited good, if any at all, and decided that it was a costly luxury which they could easily dispense with. Taking the waters was, of course, a completely un-medical approach to the problem of relieving aches and pains. If it worked it probably did so psychologically because of patients' conviction of its potency. Patients who go to the modern Tunbridge Wells spa are normally directed by their friends and relatives who may have benefited from the treatment or by their family doctors. At Bath, visitors may spend a few hours in the pleasant Pump Room, occasionally drinking from the nearby spring. But, although they may enjoy a rest in pleasant surroundings, there is little supervision nowadays either there or at any remaining spa in Britain. They are now mostly places in which to enjoy a period of convalescence and recuperate from serious illness.

5 A bridegroom of ninety-three

Many villages in the Caucasus region of the USSR are so high up that people rarely look overhead to see clouds; they look down instead. The clouds float by through the gorges below like fleets of majestic white ships. The air of the mountain villages is unpolluted, clear and cold like living crystal. The Caucasian villagers feel that they live in the borderland between Heaven and Earth.

The two men from the foothills got down from a dusty and dented bus after a steep, serpentine journey up to the village of Kikuni in Daghestan, one of the most mountainous states in the world. One was employed by the Soviet newspaper *Daghestanskaya Pravda*. His name was Alexander Grach. His companion was a gerontologist (specialist in ageing) called Ramazan Alikishi.

They had come to see the oldest woman in the whole state, perhaps in the whole of the Caucasus. She was reputed to be 160 years of age . . . with not much longer to go. So it was important to see her soon. But the meeting would not be yet because they had first to see the giant, Osman Abdurakh-manov. Osman was no stranger to them. He was well-known for his screen roles as a ferocious pirate or robber and was also renowned as a wrestler. Alikishi had already asked Osman to be their guide and to introduce them to other people in the highlands of Daghestan.

Grach was expecting a big man; but he was none the less astonished when confronted by Osman, who was more than seven feet tall, and brawny with it. Grach recorded in an article he wrote for his newspaper:

When we entered the courtyard we saw Osman by the light of the small electric bulb on the lamp-post. Perhaps it was only the play of light and shade but I could have sworn he was bigger than the lamp-post. I held out my hand and the next moment I felt it engulfed in a palm that was stretched down to me. Our host then took us by our elbows and gently propelled us towards the house, but I felt he could just as easily have lifted us up and carried us.

The visitors had arrived late and retired to bed soon after supper, knowing that it was Osman's habit to get up at five o'clock in the morning. They were awakened at that hour by the clatter of dishes (and the sound of their host singing in a deep and sonorous voice), to find Osman and his wife preparing breakfast.

Osman, with his large white, upturned moustache, 'like the wings of a soaring seagull', seemed if anything bigger than he had the night before. He was well over eighty, he told his visitors, but some of his neighbours called him 'boy' because he was not yet a hundred like most of themselves. Osman also told them that he was never ill; had perfect sight and hearing and his regular diet included milk, green vegetables, lean meats and fruit juice or fruit. He drank very little alcohol and had recently given up smoking.

After breakfast he led Grach and Ramazan Alikishi out into the bright sunlight and heady, pine-scented air to walk to the neighbouring village of Levashi to take part in the

March festival of Ploughing the First Furrow. When they arrived, Grach recalled, pipes were playing and drums beating. Everything was being done according to tradition. And these mountaineers were dowsing each other with cold mountain water, the symbol of happiness and fertility.

'The merry-making began on the outskirts of the village,' he wrote. 'First, an unusual procession moved across a field. It was headed by two bullocks hauling a wooden plough. A horse and a harrow followed, while a powerful caterpillar tractor brought up in the rear . . . living agricultural history.'

The sports of the day included horse-racing, wrestling and stone throwing with very heavy stones. Rather like 'putting the shot'. The most exciting event was the sprint. Certainly it was most unusual by Western standards because, of the twenty men who took part in the race, the youngest was eighty and the oldest was 104. What is more, the sprinters had bare feet, though the ground was covered with a layer of snow.

The umpire waved his flag and the race began with the eighty-year-old taking the lead, but a few seconds later he was overtaken by the oldest competitor, who stayed ahead to the finishing-line. 'As he came puffing in,' wrote Grach, 'dozens of hands snatched him and tossed him into the air.' The umpire then presented him with a loaf of Caucasian bread specially baked for the occasion. Those who came second and third got smaller loaves.

Grach went on, 'Two old men sitting next to me shook their heads, regretting that Habbib, a 93-year-old collective farmer who had won the race the previous year had not been able to take part. He happened to be away "on his honeymoon".'

From Levashi, Osman, the towering film actor escorted the journalist and the gerontologist to Kaka-Makhi. Until then the really old people they had met had been men, but in Kaka-Makhi they were introduced to many women who were a hundred years old or more.

For instance, there was Ashura Talmenova who reckoned she had lived for 146 years, and Hava Gazieva who said she had just celebrated her 126th birthday. Neither had ever known ill health. And then there were the Bagandov sisters, who chattered at such length and so quickly that Grach had his work cut out to record a fraction of it. Hamis Bagandov was a mere 117 and Hadiyat even younger. Hadiyat recalled that long, long ago her parents had tried to force her into marriage with a khan but she had resisted, even though it caused a social storm at the time.

It seemed that Hadiyat had indeed been lucky to have her way for, as Grach reported: 'Old men in these parts are not to be argued with. A son does not sit down in the presence of his father until he has permission to do so. He does not dare to put in a word while his father is speaking. This is one of the laws of the mountain people and these laws are never broken. When an old man enters an office everyone rises, no matter what his position ... In this area there is a large number of 130–140 year-olds. Most of them work looking after sheep, gathering firewood, some even hunting.'

*

High in the mountains, Alikishi received a letter which had been following him by mail. It contained an invitation for himself and his companions to attend a wedding in the village of Sulevkent and was signed by Ahmed Adamov and Manna Aliyeva. The invitation was unusual because weddings in Daghestan generally take place in late Autumn when the harvests from fields and orchards have been gathered and, stranger still, the gerontologist could not remember having met either Ahmed or Manna. There was no question, however, of declining the invitation – it would have been too great an insult.

The village of Sulevkent, with its clusters of two-storey wooden houses clinging to hillside slopes, is on the other side of Daghestan, but by taking a helicopter trip and hitching several car and lorry rides, the three men arrived there in about twenty-four hours – just in time.

The villagers were all dressed in their best; the men in great shaggy Astrakhan hats and long felt cloaks, the women with brightly coloured shawls over their dresses. All were walking gaily down the street towards a house from which came the beat of drums. Under the trees in the courtyard stood a long wooden table at the head of which sat an old man and an old woman. Alikishi, who had made enquiries on the journey, whispered to Grach, 'It's not an ordinary wedding . . . it's a "super-golden wedding" . . . Ahmed and Manna are actually celebrating the hundredth anniversary of their marriage.'

Now, Grach said, he understood why a gerontologist had been invited. Hundredth anniversaries did not happen every day, even in the Caucasus.

The toastmaster rose from his seat and proposed a toast that all present might share the honour and happiness befitting the occasion; after which the journalist wrote: 'No sooner had I emptied my glass than the next toast was proposed, this one to the health of Ahmed's and Manna's relatives. It turned out that this applied to everybody at the table except ourselves. They were all relatives. Many were the couple's children, grandchildren and great-grandchildren.

'The guests drank wine while the two central figures sipped

tea. Then the dancing began and Ahmed drew the stick. (According to custom the person who gets the stick dances in the centre of the circle. Later he passes it on to another who has to take his place.) The drum-beating grew louder and louder as a young girl in white glided smoothly towards Ahmed, who took a few steps and then, suddenly, turned into a whirlwind. I could not believe my eyes ... This man was unquestionably 126 years old.'

The celebrations went on far into the night.

A few days later Grach and the gerontologist, having said good-bye to Osman, set out for the village of Khutrakh to visit the old woman of 160 who was near the end of her life. By this time, Grach wrote, he had the fanciful impression that the world was populated by old people. But perhaps 'old age' was a term without real meaning here. There was life, consistently vigorous, healthy life; and it might be long or short. Old age might be a conventional concept but these peoples, who really enjoyed long life and vitality, could forget about it.

The old woman's name was Tsurba. She had apparently lived twice as long as most of the fittest people in the world normally do. Tsurba was very small, so small indeed that she was lying in a baby's cradle – ending her life where she had started it. There was no pain or suffering in her eyes, said Grach. She was evidently aware that she was dying but had no fear of death.

'Some oldtimers,' he wrote, 'told us that when Tsurba reached 140 years of age she began to shrink. Nobody had ever heard her complain about her health. She had simply withered away like an old tree. But since it was completely natural it was no longer a tragedy. To healthy people old age approaches slowly and imperceptibly. The organism gradually ceases to function; even the instinct for life fades, and finally comes death . . . as welcome as sleep.'

*

Astan Shlarba, the story goes, was rather put out. He had wanted to show off his new horse to some visitors from the West, and sent his son to bring the animal round from the paddock. His son, however, had bungled the job and had lost control of the horse, a rather fiery creature, and let it escape. Now he had returned alone, dusty and shamefaced. So Astan had to go and recapture the horse himself. The story seems to have pretty commonplace features until you know that the son was in his fifties at the time and Astan himself was a vigorous 123.

The Shlarba family live in the tobacco hamlet of Dzerba, Georgia, the main tobacco- and wine-producing state of the Caucasus. The inhabitants are said to include one-third of the Soviet Union's twenty-one thousand centenarians. They are a tough lot, with something of the self-confidence – not to say arrogance – of Texans, tending to feel independent of the rest of the USSR. For example, they resolutely decline to remove the statue of Stalin (himself a Georgian) that stands high in the centre of their capital city, Tbilisi.

It was at Dzerba, however, that the visitors from the West, a reporting team from the *Sunday Times* colour supplement, made their first port of call and met Astan, whom they found to be specially popular in the village and the first man to be consulted on matters of importance locally. The visitors reported later that although Astan tended to be forgetful concerning recent events, he could remember in detail things which had happened a long time ago. He gave them a vivid account of how he escaped from the Turks when they raided Georgia in 1920.

Although many other villagers had television, Astan had firmly turned his face from it, preferring to relax over a drink with his neighbour Sharmat, a mere 101-year-old. The visitors found the two old chaps sitting on Astan's large verandah playing the tari (Georgia's version of the mandolin). What they were doing, it transpired, was rehearsing for a forth-coming concert to be given by the local orchestra to which they belonged – and to which only centenarians could belong.

Further up in the mountains was the tea-growing village of Lyxny which has a celebrated Council of Elders which, again, consists only of men who are over a hundred years old. The council advises on local affairs, including the efficient running of the tea factory, and deals with petty crimes. The senior member of the council was then a farmer named Senat Dzeniye aged 120. He told the visitors that his family num-bered fifty, including an eldest son of ninety-five. That even-ing the visitors were entertained to dinner of roast chicken, goat and a kind of porridge made from maize, like the *polenta* of the Far East, which originated in India. They also drank innumerable toasts in grape vodka.

Later, the *Sunday Times* reporters commented: 'For all their open-handedness the Georgians are not very communicative about their longevity. They regard it as a matter of course. For instance, when we found 140-year-old Vanno Djachadzi at work outside the village of Telavi, he was at first distinctly annoyed at having to break off from pruning his vines to answer what he clearly regarded as ridiculous questions about his age.'

Vanno was one of the few Georgians they met who had

spent any length of time away from the village. He told them how he had run away from home at the age of twelve and made his way to the former St Petersburg by stowing away on Volga barges and scrounging lifts on farm carts. Back in 1917 he had helped storm the Tbilisi bank for the Bolsheviks, only settling down at home after the Revolution. The visitors did not have an opportunity to meet Shirali Muslimov, since he lived in the neighbouring state of Azerbaydzhan, but they heard much about him from the peoples of Georgia.

Shirali was then reported to be 160, certainly the oldest man in the Soviet Union and most probably the oldest man in the world. The Georgians had no difficulty in believing that Shirali was that age, and still working. Given the right circumstances, including unpolluted air, fresh and well-balanced food, plenty of exercise, reasonable temperance and good family ties ... well, anyone might do it.

6 'Old men are liars!'

The outside world first began to hear about Shirali Muslimov in late 1966, when he came down from the mountain village of Barzavu for a medical check-up at Baku, the capital of Azerbaydzhan. For, on that occasion, only the second time he had visited Baku, Shirali consented to appear at a press conference. It was a jolly affair with the old man, lean and with a bushy beard, joking with his questioners. He had declined an opportunity, his first ever, to ride in a private motor-car, but had thoroughly enjoyed travelling in a tram.

A few months earlier Shirali had celebrated his 161st birthday and had also been decorated with the Order of the Red Banner of Labour, awarded for his lifetime work as a fruit farmer. He told newspaper men that the doctors who had just examined him had found him in perfect health.

Asked the inevitable questions about how he had managed to live so long the old man said that one reason was that he had made it a lifelong rule never to hurry – he certainly wasn't in a hurry to die! He said he got up every day at sunrise; kept to a correctly balanced diet; said his prayers and worked several hours in the orchard he had laid out himself a hundred years earlier. His father, he said, had lived to be more than 120 years and his mother to 110.

Three years after that visit to Baku, Shirali Muslimov was

made the 'star' of a film about the old people of Azerbaydzhan which spread his fame still further – at least in the Soviet Union. And, from that time, every Muslimov birthday became a big event, with crowds of curious visitors climbing the mountains to pay their respects to the patriarch of Barzavu. When the film was released, it was said that there were almost a hundred centenarians to every hundred thousand of the population of Azerbaydzhan. Featured with Muslimov in the film were Hanlar Guseinov aged 127 and his 97-year-old wife Salata-Hala. They had recently celebrated their diamond wedding anniversary. The film commentary was spoken by Shirin Gazanov from the village of Chereken – who at the time was himself almost 150 years old.

Gazanov died four years later and it was reported that he had been working out-of-doors up to the last few days. The astonishing Shirali, however, was still alive and well and living in Barzavu where he had spent almost every day since he was born. On Shirali's 167th birthday the Moscow news agency, Novosti, reported that he had danced the lively *lezghinka* along with his grandsons Murzagusein, aged eighty-eight, and Muslim, aged seventy-one. That year Shirali also celebrated the seventy-fifth anniversary of his marriage to his third wife; and a baby girl called Sevindzh was born to his great grand-daughter, Taji – the 215th member of the Muslimov family.

Even on his 167th birthday in 1972, Novosti reported, Shirali Muslimov drank only lemonade to toast his guests. The report added: 'Shirali has never drunk alcohol or smoked. He puts the source of his long life down to the fact that he has worked since childhood and has led a healthy open-air life. And he has lived all his life in the mountains. When he was younger he was considered one of the best horsemen in the area and he stopped riding only very recently.'

When the end came for Shirali Muslimov in September 1973, just after his 168th birthday, it came with great peace and dignity. The old man had taken to his bed, feeling more than usually tired, and the next day the tiredness was still with him. Relatives, the old and young, came and stood by him, speaking in whispers and waiting for what they knew was inevitable. It was not a time for lamentation, hardly even for sadness. It was a time for wonder: that a man should have lived so long and ailed so little. And when Shirali ceased to breathe it seemed not so much that he had died but that life had quietly withdrawn from him.

*

As mentioned earlier there are other places – not only within the Soviet Union, like Abkhazia, Uzbekistan, Yakutia and Altay, for example – but in other parts of the world such as Ecuador and Hunza in the Himalayas, where people live to spectacular ages. But before dealing with them let us consider for a moment the views of a man – and a Russian at that – who is highly suspicious and sceptical about the stories emerging from the Caucasus region, views which were summed up unequivocally in the *Sunday Times* headline OLD MEN ARE LIARS.

Dr Zhoras Medvedev is a biochemist and gerontologist. Having been deprived of his Soviet citizenship in 1973, following criticism of Russia's postal service and censorship of international correspondence, he now works at the National Institute for Medical Research, London. In October 1974 Dr Medvedev had an article published in the American journal – *The Gerontologist* – which stated that despite intensive research no scientific explanations had yet been found to account for peaks of longevity in the Caucasus and other areas of the Soviet Union famous for their old people.

'The most common approach, which was popular for a long time – the influence of special conditions in mountain areas – proved to be invalid after investigation into details of the geographical distribution of super-longevity,' Dr Medvedev wrote; meaning to say that it was wrong to suppose you could only find old people living on mountain tops in ideal climatic conditions.

He went on: 'In Yakutia and Altay Plain areas the climate is extremely cold, dry and continental. Ecuador has a tropical climate. In the Caucasus areas the climate has all possible variations: humid and subtropical in Abkhazia . . . dry and more continental in Central Georgia and Azerbaydzhan.

'In large, relatively flat areas of the North Caucasus the climate is roughly similar to the so-called corn belt of the USA. There is no evident correlation between longevity and mountain level, even in Georgia. There are some places at sea-level with a higher index of longevity than the nearest mountain regions and the distribution of this index between mountain populations at equal altitudes is very wide . . .' (In other words it has been found that in some places there were more very old people living at sea-level than in the mountains.)

Medvedev's interest in the phenomenon of extreme old age was aroused when he was still a student living in Tbilisi. He had been fascinated by reports published by the Russian gerontologist Bogomoletz and his colleagues, following an expedition to Georgia in 1937 organized by the Kiev Institute of Clinical Physiology to study the health of a large group of centenarians.

'Bogomoletz,' wrote Medvedev, 'was the main expert on problems of ageing in the USSR and was very enthusiastic about the possibility of experimental prolongation of human life. Reports on this expedition were published in the form of a collection of case records of centenarians aged 110 to 150 years but, in almost every case, Bogomoletz established the fact that no reliable documents establishing ages existed and that these people were not as old as they claimed to be.' (It has since been pointed out by Soviet gerontologists and Neil Lyall that church records as well as inter-state passports of Czarist days gave fairly reliable records of dates of birth.)

'Bogomoletz,' wrote Medvedev, 'usually did not believe the highest age claims (120 to 160 years) but he nevertheless believed that all these people were at least centenarians.'

If the old people of the Caucasus and elsewhere do tend to exaggerate their ages slightly, is there any reason for doing so other than failure to take proper account of the passing years? Another Soviet scientist, Berdyshev, who studied the longevity problem in the mountains of South Altay, puts forward the notion that they may have been prompted by a desire to achieve greater authority.

Medvedev also took this line with regard to the Caucasians, saying: 'The older a person is the more respect and honour he (or she) receives. Centenarians are usually chairmen of local councils, celebrations, dinners, marriages and other functions. The most elderly people are almost regarded as saints. Such traditions create the stimulus to exaggerate age a little, especially when there are no living witnesses to remember when the "oldest person in the village" was really born . . .'

Medvedev also put this view: 'Local honour and publicity surrounding centenarians has been supplemented during recent decades by publicity at district, regional, republican and even all-Union levels by articles, pictures in newspapers and magazines, by interviews, by special medical attention, etc.'

He pointed out that longevity records were, somewhat surprisingly, climbing all the time. During the 1940s they reached 130 and 140 years and now several persons are considered to be as old as 160 to 170 years.

Finally, Medvedev alleged that the Soviet Union had 'seized upon the legendary longevity of its peoples for propaganda purposes'. This led to statements such as 'The Soviet Union is the country with the record longevity of human beings . . . The number of centenarians is increasing parallel with our approach to the creation of a Communist Society.'

In this connection it is perhaps worth mentioning that the Soviet Ministry of Posts and Communications, which came into being in 1956, issued a special postage stamp depicting one of the then oldest citizens of the USSR. He was Makhmoud Fivazov of Daghestan and at the time his age was said to be 148 years. However, Ramazan Alikishi, already mentioned, who studied longevity in Daghestan over a long period, declared that the average age of the men he examined was 111.5 years and that of the women 115.4 years . . . which presupposes that not a few of both sexes were very considerably older. And Dr Grigory Pitskelauri, the Gerontological Institute's doctor in Tbilisi, also seems to have faith in the sincerity of his super-centenarians, to say nothing of his admiration for their life-style. They have always lived extremely regular lives, he says, rising at the same early hour every day, taking three or four meals daily and retiring early to bed. All the four hundred cases he studied in Georgia were of average intelligence or higher, and remarkably stable emotionally.

Only eight of these had not brought up large families. A Tass Agency report of the doctor's work made it clear that he, at any rate, favoured the good, unpolluted air and high-altitude theory. Nearly all Pitskelauri's subjects, it was stated, lived more than five thousand feet up and they had worked hard during their younger days. Sixty per cent of them were still working.

'Most of the old people,' he said, 'do not smoke. Their diet consists of traditional peppery Georgian food, and they eat a lot of vegetables and fruit, lean meat, milk, cheese and un-strained honey. Such diseases as cancer and tuberculosis are very rare indeed among them.'

It is also worth mentioning that the observers sent to Georgia for the feature in a *Sunday Times* colour supplement, which included a number of photographs of the mountain people, evidently had no difficulty in accepting that they were the ages they claimed to be. The way the colour supplement put it was this:

'There can be no real doubt of their age despite the absence of early nineteenth-century birth certificates. The Soviet Institutes of Gerontology have subjected them to years of study which have really not been coloured by any sort of medical nationalism. And, apart from the scientific evidence, it is a highly convincing experience to hear, say, 140-year-old Vanno Djachiadzi from Telavi village describing the scandal in St Petersburg (now Leningrad) in 1837, when Pushkin was sensationally murdered by his wife's lover in a rigged duel.'

Many Soviet Institutes of Gerontology have maintained accurate records of the long-livers in the USSR (including authenticated dates of birth). World-famous medical research centres, like the Institute of Gerontology at Kiev, Geronto-logical Institutes at Baku and Tbilisi, the Metchnikov centres at Odessa and others have authenticated many of these great ages.

But, before drawing any firm conclusions let us take a trip to the other side of the world, to another area where people are said to live a very long time in an enviable state of health and vitality.

7 Marviloso!

During the rainy season many of the primitive roads across the Andes mountains are regularly washed away. Heavy deluges obliterate every trace of them, especially those which are little more than tracks anyway.

The bus from Quito groaned and spluttered its way up to the provincial capital of Loja with a dozen or so chattering passengers wearing wide-brimmed hats and colourful shawls. Among them sat a slim, pale-faced man from London. Dr David Davies, a member of the Gerontology Unit at London University, was enjoying the drive; the scenery enthralled him and he had a growing sense of excitement about what lay ahead.

In an account of the journey which appeared in the doctors' newspaper *On Call* in May 1973, Dr Davies said the bus went only as far as Loja, after which he'd had to wait until the next day to complete the journey in a clapped-out jeep – travelling a further fifty kilometres. This was the worst part. The driver and his passenger frequently had to get down from the jeep to repair the road before they could go any further.

Dr Davies wrote: 'Ever since I'd left Quito three days earlier the sky had been overcast, the rain heavy and frequent. But suddenly as the jeep lurched and slithered round yet another hairpin bend there lay before us a lovely, sun-drenched valley – Vilcabamba.'

The valley, Dr Davies found, was not unlike some of those in Southern Germany. It was about ten kilometres long by six and a half kilometres wide (six miles by four miles) and 1,500 metres (five thousand feet) above sea level, with the temperature remaining pretty constant around 19 degrees Centigrade (66 degrees Fahrenheit). But it was the people who interested him most, for he had heard from leading doctors in Quito that some of the Vilcabambans were well into their second century. And the important thing from a scientific standpoint was that their ages could be authenticated because they were all of Spanish descent and had baptismal certificates to support their claims to unusual longevity.

'This is not always the case,' wrote Dr Davies. 'Too often claims to great age are quite impossible to substantiate with any degree of certainty; after a time it becomes a source of pride, memories become hazy, contemporaries die, and it is all too easy to add a year or two to the correct age without anyone really noticing!'

Any qualms he may have had in accepting that the Vilcàbambans were as old as they said were evidently dispelled during a subsequent visit to Ecuador, for in *Modern Geriatrics*, published in February 1975, he commented:

Last year we found one village which has records going back to 1665. In most of the villages concerned, the records go back to the eighteenth century at least ... The parish registers give information on births, marriages and deaths and indicate that the phenomenon of old age in the region is nothing new.

'There are eighteenth-century records of people dying aged 150 and a priest (for it was the priests who kept the registers and who

62

were probably the only literate or semi-literate members of the community) had written in the margin beside one such entry, in now faded ink, *Marviloso*!'

Dr Davies said it was not known how many centenarians were living in the Vilcabamba valley and other villages of Ecuador but in one village he had found at least three men who were all over 132. He added,

'In these villages they do not understand the meaning of old age – at least not in the way we do. I have frequently been asked, "Do you not have people living to 120 and 130 in London?" Within their own communities they are not in any way considered unusual, particularly as none are infirm and all can in some way contribute to the community. Indeed, the only person I saw hobbling around on crutches was a man of twenty-six who had injured his toe playing football!

'Nearly all the people of these villages are lean and athletic looking. There is no obesity to be seen, and most are of medium height. The men, in particular, keep a good head of hair to the end of their days . . . Many seem to have a bright sparkle in their eyes which adds to their appearance of liveliness.

'Some of the old men . . . claim that it's love that keeps them going so well. What we do know is that they have very large families, are said to have fertile sperm until a remarkably late age, and that cancer is unknown in these valleys.'

Dr Davies concluded his *Modern Geriatrics* report by saying:

'The discovery of these people must come as a great shock to the North American social structure – which is generally geared to age-group systems and the general expectation of a fairly rapid and in-evitable ageing after, say, forty years – to see and hear about these cheerful, lithe and agile people of around the ninety or a hundred mark . . . These people not only have interesting tales to tell us, but they can help us repair and improve our own lives; provided, of course, that we allow ourselves a little time in which to discover what makes them tick for such a remarkably long span.'

In Vilcabamba, he found, it was common to encounter people aged a hundred years or more carrying on as though they were only half that age. The oldest inhabitant was José David who, at the time, was 142 years old. Then there was Miguel Carpio, a mere 123 years of age. José David was busy hoeing around his vegetables and Miguel Carpio was also working. There was no doubt whatever about their ages. Both these men had documentary proof in the form of baptismal certificates.

The remarkable thing about the old people of Vilcabamba is their activity. Most of them live on scattered farms and smallholdings which are largely self supporting and everyone takes his turn with the work. When first seen by the visitor from London José David's face was tanned and weather-beaten.

All the Vilcabambans, said Dr Davies, seem to retain their alertness and normal faculties until the time of their death. And all seem to have some role to fulfil. This, in itself, is most interesting and suggests something we are only just beginning to realize – that a feeling of usefulness really does contribute to health, both mental and physical, in elderly people.

Dr Davies remarked: 'The diet of the valley's peoples is very simple and might well be a lesson to us. The consumption of calories is very low . . . at an average of 1500 to 1700 per head of the adult population per day it is about half the intake in Britain. The diet is largely based on fresh fruit and vege-

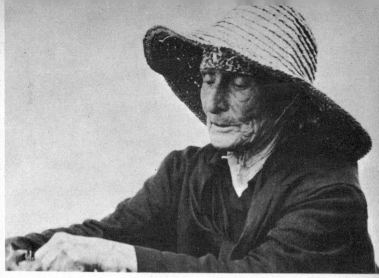

Above Until she died in 1975, aged 139 years, Mrs Khfaf Lazuria was thought to be the oldest woman in the world. She lived in Kutol, Abkhazia where she worked on the tea plantations. *Below* Balashki and Anina Orendjeo are both over 125 years old and in splendid health. This picture was taken to celebrate their 100th wedding anniversary with hot drinks from the samovar.

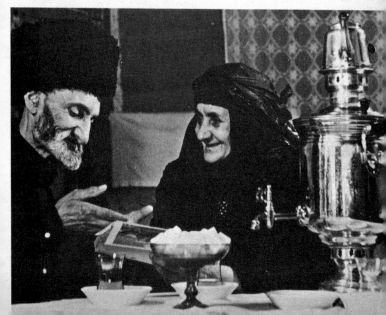

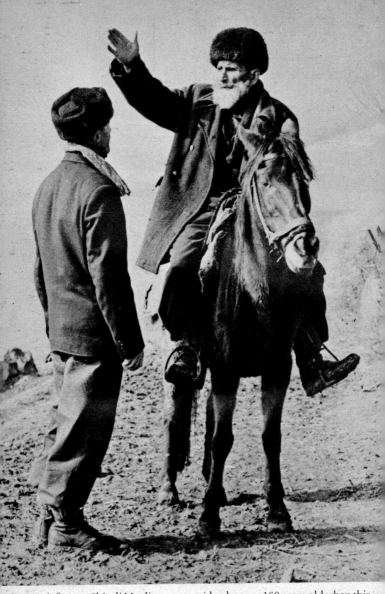

Fruit farmer Shirali Muslimov was said to be over 160 years old when this picture was taken near the mountain village of Barzavu in Azerbaydzhan.

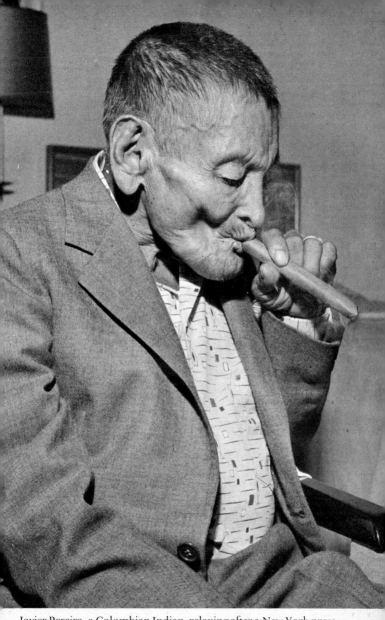

Javier Pereira, a Colombian Indian, relaxing after a New York press conference in 1950. He was more than 160 years old at the time and was 4ft 4in high.

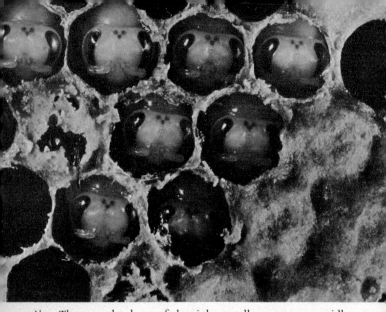

Above The young bee larvae, fed mainly on pollen, grow very rapidly and are soon ready to leave their cells. *Below* This worker bee heads for the hive with its quota of nectar (for conversion into honey) and two large loads of bee-collected pollen adhering to the hairs on its legs.

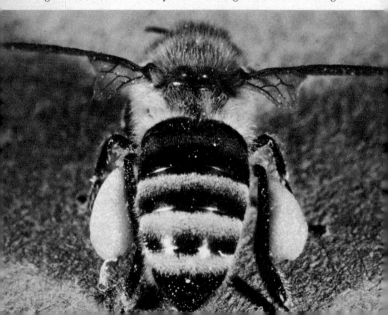

tables, mostly grown in their own gardens, with only lean meat and little or no animal fat. Not many cows are kept and what milk there is is turned almost entirely into cheese.'

Meals are frugal by our standards, consisting mainly of soup made from sweetcorn, yuke (a root), potato and beans. There are several varieties of beans and oranges which are grown locally. Lean meat (without any animal fat) is eaten but is always accompanied by green home-grown vegetables. Sweetness, apart from the fruit, is provided by crude, unstrained honey (its cloudiness being due to a high proportion of pollen) and unrefined sugar cane which the valley people grow themselves in small quantities. Their diet is, therefore, free from refined carbohydrates and is, most definitely, free from many of the over-refined, dietarily unnecessary foods which we ourselves so disastrously take for granted. No 'processed' foods are eaten; fancy cakes and pastries are unknown and so, too, are pies, sausages and 'sweet confectionery' – like toffees, chocolates and fancy biscuits. A type of crispbread is popular.

What is surprising, however, according to Dr Davies's report, is that Vilcabambans, especially the older ones, all tend to drink and smoke heavily. Swallowing between two and four cups of rum a day and smoking up to sixty or even eighty cigarettes daily is considered nothing unusual. But before starting to question our own beliefs about these habits it should be remembered that, although their rum is fairly potent, it is home-made and their cigarettes are also rolled individually from tobacco grown in local gardens. Says Dr Davies: 'The cigarettes are rolled in maize leaves (though toilet paper is preferred if it is obtainable). Also, as the cigarettes are rolled by hand the tobacco content of each is fairly low. But, as with their diets, these things are unrefined and have no additives to improve appearance or shelf life. They do not have to compete in an overcrowded consumer market, and any additives are always natural products.

'The older generation also swear by herbal teas, though these are inevitably laughed at by the younger generation as superstitious nonsense. I frequently saw the older ladies collecting these herbs and plants from river banks. An infusion is also made from the local herbs to which is attributed health and life-giving properties, too.'

Vilcabamba has a gentle climate and the people talk of the tranquillity of their valley. Few of them have ever left it even to travel as far as Loja – twenty-five miles away. They work and sleep and relax in the sun; they very rarely quarrel; they never concern themselves with the frenetic outside world. But, as in the case of their contemporaries in other parts of the world, especially the Soviet Union, there seems to be some mystery in the Vilcabambans' ability to survive so long. Is it due to diet, genetic factors, trace elements in the soil or the water or what?

Since Dr Davies's first visit in 1971 there has been an almost continuous medical and anthropological assault on Vilcabamba, aimed at discovering exactly what makes the valley people tick, and go on ticking so consistently. But if there is irrefutable proof that some of the Vilcabambans do live up to half-way through their second century, surely this is an added reason to suppose that the same may be true of the Himalayans and the peoples of the Caucasus. And if they can do it – and scientists seem to agree that it has nothing to do with the climate – then why not the rest of us . . . the British and Americans, the French, Germans, Italians, Dutch, Spanish,

Austrians, Scandinavians, Australasians, Eskimos – the whole lot?

It does seem that the life-style of all these long-livers and their regimens of living and eating have many things in common. Unpolluted air is undoubtedly a most desirable feature and city-dwellers in general suffer more strains and stresses than those who live in rural areas. Other features – such as diet, exercise and regular periods of rest – are all-important.

*

But let us reconsider for a moment the conditions in Ecuador and Azerbaydzhan, where living sky-high ensures a good supply of unpolluted air. Paradoxically, the life-giving gas, oxygen, is relatively scarce at higher altitudes. But is it possible that living and working at a high altitude in some way or another enables the human heart to work more efficiently?

Professor Pierre Moret, secretary-general of the International Society of Cardiology based in Geneva, is an eminent physician who believes that it does. He led an expedition into the Andes to investigate the stout-heartedness of the Andeans and concluded that their heart action was more efficient than that of people living at sea level. He has been working on a theory that there is a special adaptive mechanism which not only compensates for oxygen scarcity but also makes the heart physically more rugged at high altitudes. He reckons that all of us are born with this mechanism but the vast majority lose it in early infancy. This action has nothing to do with blood circulation, says Professor Moret, but seems to be fundamental to the cellular structure of heart muscles. The professor and his team have demonstrated the existence of this mechanism with laboratory rats taken 500 metres

(1,500 feet) up in the Swiss Alps. After six months, tests showed that the rats' hearts had undergone a subtle change, enabling them to adapt to life at a higher altitude, and all the rats seemed healthier for it. It cannot be assumed, however, that human hearts would adapt in the same way – a good deal more research is needed. So Professor Moret does not advise anyone – especially if he has a weak heart – to take to the hills just yet.

*

Dr Davies, in his article in *On Call* made the point that the Vilcabamba diet, which includes a good deal of fresh fruit and vegetables, is low in animal fat. This is significant because of a growing conviction among doctors and dieticians all over the world that animal fat plays an ugly part in the death toll from heart disease in the Western world. Between them they have produced a grim kind of league table showing the extent to which heart disease plagues different countries.

At the top of the table, rather surprisingly, comes Finland. This vigorous nation of barely 4,500,000 is renowned for its strong, open-air people who, on the face of it, should be the last to suffer from coronary attacks. Indeed, it used to be something of a medical mystery – but not so much since Professor Osmo Turpeinen, a leading Helsinki research scientist, and his colleagues, produced a remarkable paper* on Finland's heart troubles.

Heart attacks are commonly thought to be due to heavy smoking, high blood pressure and over-indulgence in rich foods. The affluent society has long been indicted as the overall culprit. But the Finns have never been particularly

*Published in the *Lancet*

affluent. This is what intrigued the Finnish researchers. So, back in 1958, they started planning an experiment aimed at solving the mystery, particularly the part played by certain foodstuffs in producing cholesterol, a substance that causes the 'furring up' and eventual clogging of arteries.

The Finns worked out two diet sheets which, although they looked identical, were not. One consisted of normal food such as most of us eat regularly, the other of foods containing much more of what is known by the ungainly term 'polyunsaturated fats' and less of animal fats. Over the next twelve years, hundreds of Finns (none of whom knew they were taking part in an experiment) were given one or the other of these diets and records were kept of their health.

The people, mostly middle-aged and of both sexes, were all long-term patients at two Helsinki hospitals, known for the experiment only by the initial letters 'N' and 'K'.

For the first six years the selected group in hospital 'N' were given the test diet and those in hospital 'K' the ordinary diet. Then, for a further six years, the diets were switched round. Both diets were, of course, equally good from a general nutritional point of view but what Turpeinen and his team did in the case of the test diet was to cut out meat fat and use vegetable oil exclusively for cooking. The patients' egg ration was reduced; milk was skimmed of cream and emulsified with soya bean oil. Besides this, butter and ordinary margarine were replaced by 'soft' margarine with a high content of polyunsaturated fats.

At the end of the first six-year period the incidence of heart attacks among patients on the test diet was about half that of those on the ordinary diet. And at the end of the second six-year period after the diets had been switched, the incidence of heart attacks among patients was again about half that of patients on an ordinary diet. Routine tests showed that test-diet patients had much lower cholesterol levels in their blood. These 'blind' tests were decisive and it was clearly established that the use of vegetable fats and the avoidance of animal fats was an effective method of preventing many heart troubles. Asked about Finland's unenviable place at the head of the coronary league table, Turpeinen said later, 'I think we are getting what we deserve. It seems we eat too much animal fat and probably our drinking – and smoking – habits are partly to blame as well.'

Lapland, Finland, Poland, Latvia and many North European countries where 'speck' is widely eaten also suffer from jaundice and other liver ailments. 'Speck' is the fat trimmed off bacon and is eaten with bread in considerable quantities.

*

Recently, scientists have more or less agreed that a low calorie diet and the reduction of animal fats including butter are essential factors in the attainment of longevity. Animal fats, including cream, can be replaced with vegetable oils which contribute towards longevity . . . and freedom from heart troubles and stomach upsets. Again, it does not seem that cigars and cheroots are so harmful as cigarettes nor does it appear that a sweet sherry occasionally or a bottle of wine with meals is likely to do any harm.

Cream should be avoided as well as butter. Soft margarine is a much healthier item of diet, containing, as it does, vegetable oils.

An inquiry into the diet of the Finnish people, particularly those living in North Karelia, showed that no less than 39 per cent of their diet consisted of fats, including 22 per cent of animal fat. Even in America, where heart disease is a serious national problem, though at last it seems to be declining, the diet includes 18 per cent of animal fat. In countries lower down the coronary-risk scale it may be less than 12 per cent.

'I think,' concluded Turpeinen, 'my colleagues and myself are justified in saying that cutting down on fatty foods that produce cholesterol will at least delay the onset of heart attacks. We do not claim to have the complete answer to coronary disease but there is evidence now that dietary habits are changing in Finland, especially among the more educated people.'

It is reported elsewhere in this book that nobody ever died of sheer old age, but, rather, against a background of diseases of old age including heart troubles, arteriosclerosis, blood pressure, bronchial pneumonia, cancer and serious over-weight. At least two of these fatal ailments can be avoided by the replacement of vegetable oils for animal fats – which it is suggested should be avoided wherever possible. Any excess of fats, sugar, common salt and sauces or seasoning, cream and sweet confectionery should also be avoided in the search for restored youthfulness and vitality. All such items must be eaten very sparsely. Like the researches on animal fats, they have all been carefully investigated, and the results of avoiding risks can be very worthwhile indeed.

8 A diet of apricots

The notion that ideal circumstances might enable people to live far beyond the normal span was splendidly exploited by James Hilton in his best-selling novel, *Lost Horizon*, more than forty years ago. Hilton wrote of an almost inaccessible valley called 'Shangri-la', hidden among the snow-peaks of the Himalayas. Shangri-la was a place of plenty, wanting nothing from the outside world. It had a perfect climate and the inhabitants lived entirely without stress, hardly giving a thought to disease and death. Such a place could not, of course, exist except between the covers of a book. Or could it?

Readers would have been surprised to learn – and may still be surprised – that the author based his story on an actual Himalayan valley where real people seemed to have discovered the secret of staying young. The valley, which is about sixty miles long and a mile or so wide, is called Hunza and its people Hunzukuts. It is practically without rainfall but Mount Pakaposhi, which towers behind the Hunza valley, is covered with eternal ice- and snow-fields and provides abundant water for domestic and irrigation purposes.

Until the eyes of the world were briefly focused on them in the early 1960s the Hunzukuts are thought to have lived in almost complete isolation for two thousand years.

One of their first visitors from the modern world was the American doctor-explorer, Dr Allen E. Banik, who later collaborated with sociologist Renee Taylor in an exciting adventure book, *Hunza Land*. In an interview for the old *Sunday Dispatch*, Dr Banik told of a hair-raising flight that took him over the mountains that cut Hunza off from the Western world:

In the aircraft, I peered through the smeared window in search of an opening . . . as we climbed steadily towards a towering range that simply had to be cleared if we were going to get in.

Under full power we just skimmed the sheer rocks, then dropped into the valley beyond. Seemingly endless peaks cast shadows over the plane as we skimmed so close to rock sides that a man on the wing could have touched them. A steep bank on the left pushed us hard into our seats as we dodged one precipitous canyon. Then, before we could get our breath in the unpressurized cabin, the Pakistani pilot made a sharp bank to the right. These pilots had no modern instruments. They flew by the seat of their pants. I strained mentally to push away the mountain that seemed about to tear off our vibrating wing. I lost five pounds before we landed.

Even after touchdown, Dr Banik said, he had a long and hazardous journey by road and only his determination to learn the secret of the fabulous Hunzukuts kept him going. He told a *Sunday Dispatch* reporter that in the valley he found men living to be 120, with all their strength and faculties. 'Some of them fathered children at the age of ninety,' he said. 'They were incredible by Western standards.'

It was all to do with the diet and life-style of these people. The women never seemed to get fat, however much they ate. And no disease had ever gained hold in the valley. 'The people

74

are too germ-resistant,' he said. 'Bugs die in contact with them.'

Dr Banik said he had learned that an average man of Hunza at the age of eighty or ninety could walk for sixty miles carrying a load and then return to his regular work immediately, without any rest. In former days messengers working for the Emir of Hunza had preferred to run rather than ride on horseback. They kept up a steady trot around the clock, stopping only briefly for short rests and food. On their return they required only their usual amount of rest.

'These men,' said Dr Banik, 'are straight and tall, broad shouldered, deep chested, slim waisted and heavy legged. They walk erect with a smooth, effortless glide that can be identified as far as it can be seen. Undoubtedly, the farming methods of the Hunzukuts and the type of food they have eaten for centuries are responsible for their remarkable vigour, long life and freedom from disease.'

Dr Banik said he was struck one day by the fact that there were no dogs in Hunza. He added, 'I noticed also that there were no cats or chickens.' His guide told him, 'Dogs need food and we do not have much of it. Cats eat mice, but we have no mice. Chickens would scratch up our fine gardens where we grow our food, so we have no chickens.'

The Hunzukuts' habit of rising early suited Dr Banik very well, for he was eager to begin his investigation into the secrets of long life and health in the valley. After enjoying a hot cup of tea he stepped out on to the verandah of the room he had been allotted. 'The air was cool, with a slight breeze,' he said. 'Men, women and children were already at their tasks. I could see cattle and sheep grazing high up the mountainsides on green patches kept lush by waters trickling down from summit snows.'

75

He learned that all Hunzukuts got up at 5 a.m., usually took a short nap in the afternoon and retired to bed at nine o'clock at night. In his book he expressed the opinion that over the centuries the citizens of the mountain state have evolved patterns of eating, living, exercising and thinking which have increased their life-span. He became convinced that diet played a fundamental part, especially in regard to their consumption of lean meat, fresh vegetables and fruit – including apricots in abundance.

The Hunzukuts' diet 'cannot be matched in our civilization, with its depleted soils, processed foods robbed of life-giving elements, and cooking methods that effectively destroy a substantial percentage of the vitamins and trace elements that are essential to sound bodies.'

It is worth adding that the Emir of Hunza, now living in retirement, strongly supported the findings of Dr Banik when he was interviewed in Paris, where he attended a wedding in October 1969. He said then that many of his ancestors had lived to be more than a hundred years old and that he himself at fifty-six had every intention of becoming a fit centenarian. The Emir said of the Western world, 'When people here reach seventy they can hardly move unless they have gone out of their way to lead healthy lives. In my country you see people working in the fields at ninety, ninety-five and even a hundred – and it is nothing for a person of ninety-five to walk ten miles a day and enjoy it.'

The Emir added, 'The reason lies in our food. We are all farmers and live on mulberries, cherries, peaches, plums, grapes and barley, but above all, apricots. Apricots are our staple diet. We eat them all the time, both raw and cooked and we use the oil from the apricot stones for cooking.' The

Hunzukuts sweetened apricots with unstrained honey.

The Hunzukuts, he said, all lived simple, happy lives. By religion they were Ismaelis. He himself was President of the Supreme Council of the Ismaeli Community (a branch of the Moslem religion), and the most venerated leader after the Aga Khan.

Apart, perhaps, from the fact that the people of Hunza have an unusually high consumption of apricots and apricot oil it does not appear that there is anything special in their diet to account for their ability to live long, healthy lives. It is not without interest, however, that Dr Banik refers to methods of cooking in which essential vitamins and trace elements are saved from destruction.

Nor can one fail to be impressed by his report on the tranquil life-style of the Hunzukuts – the same sort of life-style observed by others in Vilcabamba and the Caucasus. It seems indeed that if the total populations of these areas were to change places over night they could carry on living as happily as if they had never left home. Yet the probability is that none of these people have ever heard of the others.

What is clear is that all these long-livers are involved in one way or another with farming, and spend many hours out-of-doors. Their food is plain but fresh, though not perhaps as plentiful as the food of other countries, especially in the West. It is clear, too, that they have strong family ties and manage to get along with one another, whether related or otherwise, with the minimum aggression.

Maybe they are not clever in the intellectual sense of the word, maybe they would even be considered dim by our ophisticated standards, but it seems unquestionable that they are happier than millions elsewhere in the world. It was certainly not without pride that the Emir of Hunza told his Paris interviewer, 'In our country we have no crime, no police and no jails. The biggest punishment is exile.'

So a statement in the *Sunday Times* of 29 September 1974 came as a rather sad footnote to the story of the secluded Himalayan valley. The statement said: 'Pakistan has annexed the tiny Himalayan kingdom of Hunza, which claimed to be the model for the "perfect country" of Shangri-la in James Hilton's novel *Lost Horizon*. The take-over was announced by the Pakistan Prime Minister, Ali Bhutto, during a tour of tribal areas of his country's border with China. "Pakistan is one," Ali Bhutto said, "and cannot afford to have states within a state. It belongs to the peasants and the workers, not the princes and kings." The ruler of Hunza, Emir Jamal Khan, has been retired on pension, ending nine hundred years of feudal rule in the kingdom.'

9 Relax ... and live

Factors common to all areas where many people live well beyond the normal span of life are not difficult to detect. We have seen, for example, that the super-centenarians all breathe clean air, often in mountain districts, and there is sufficient evidence that they drink unpolluted water. What also seems unquestionable is that their diet is low in calories and animal fats that produce cholesterol – a waxy substance that in excess can cause the 'furring up' of arteries and lead to a heart attack – in the bloodstream. Even the basic *amount* of food the average centenarian consumes is relatively small by our own standards, and in some cases might be regarded as a near-starvation diet.

The old people of the Caucasus, of Hunza and Ecuador live by the sun, in the sense that they get up at dawn, work all day out-of-doors and go to bed at sunset. But is there no more to their longevity than just this regularity? Otherwise it would seem to be rather lacking in purpose, certainly in adventure.

From what we can find out about them, the long-livers do not appear to be endowed with much competitive spirit. There is nothing in their society which suggests a desire to 'keep up with the Joneses' – perhaps because the ordinary requirements of living off the land keep them too busy for such considerations. A woman wearing a new hat or shawl, for example, might arouse the interest, even the admiration, of her neighbours, but not their envy or scorn. And much the same would apply to a man with a new horse.

Crime is almost unknown because a man who does not covet his neighbour's possessions is unlikely to put himself in peril by trying to steal them, especially in a small community where the crime would soon be detected. This is not to suggest that such events never take place but that when they do the circumstances must be exceptional.

In the domains of super-centenarians a man's pride is normally confined to pride in his family, especially if it is a large family and reflects his sexual prowess – although, this, of course, is also observed in the outside world. A large family with many strong sons has been a source of human pride throughout the ages.

One thing of which the Vilcabambans, Hunzukuts and Caucasians can certainly be exonerated is the desire to get on in business that affects so many of us in the Western world; the desire to have a better car, a bigger house, a more important job; and to have them as soon as possible.

Few doctors would deny that ambition of this kind is a source of stress in many Western people and appears to be strongly associated with coronary thrombosis and death in middle-age. Family doctors are constantly advising patients to ease up, stop taking work home, to leave business problems behind in the locked office. But once one is on a collision course with heart disease, it is difficult to avoid.

Dr Hans Selye, professor and director of the Institute of Experimental Medicine and Surgery at Montreal University, Canada, has summed up the situation by saying that although the body needs a certain amount of stress, the amount must be carefully controlled. It will not hurt you, he reckons, to work hard for something you really want, but first make sure you really want it and that you have a reasonable chance of attaining it.

In an article for the medical newspaper *Pulse* in July 1975 Dr Selye was quoted thus: 'Just remember that the stress of frustration is particularly harmful. Admit that there is no perfection but in each category of achievement something is tops; be satisfied to strive for that. Whatever situation you meet in life, consider first whether it is really worth fighting for. Try to keep your mind constantly on the pleasant aspects of life and on actions which can improve your situation ...'

Above all, Dr Selye advocated: 'Do not underestimate the delight of real simplicity in your life-style ...'

This, it seems, is precisely the attitude the long-livers take (albeit unconsciously) to life. They have little or no organized sport, especially of the intensely competitive kind where even vast crowds of onlookers become emotionally involved – sometimes to the extent that they are led to cause serious damage to property and do physical harm to others in an excess of frustration or uncontrollable high spirits.

It is questionable whether organized sport, particularly competitive sport, does any good to anyone in the long term. An alternative view, again presented in *Pulse*, is that it may do positive harm to those indulging in it. The *Pulse* writer's view was:

'Sporting activites are of course traditional in school curricula. So from an early age such pursuits are encouraged and those who excel are rewarded with cups and medals. Aggression and victory at all costs are admired on the sports field, especially in the context of the team. Such activities in a different social setting would be hailed as hooliganism and sadism. Are we to be surprised at the performance of football fans whose actions are so little different from those witnessed on the field?'

The writer, a country GP, continued:

Learning, not physical training is an essential prerequisite in the sort of world in which we live. Yet I know of no evidence to show that the games activities in schools improve the examination results of the pupils. Commonsense dictates that any time spent away from the classroom can only result in poorer academic attainment. To those advocates of sport I would say that battles are no longer won on playing fields but with highly sophisticated technology.'

More to the point postulated in this book, the writer continued:

It should be appreciated by everyone, as well as doctors, that obesity is not easily controlled by exercise. After all, work all day with the energy output of an oil rigger and the result will be the loss of one pound of fat. Exercise promotes appetite beyond calorific requirements.

Dietary habits are far more important than exercise for quality of life. The proof of this, unlike exercise, is well documented. Too little food . . . and starvation results. Too much food and the sluggardly fat fall prey to heart disease. The results of an excessive animal fat intake are well known. Where is the evidence that sporting activities promote longevity and, equally important, the quality of life?

The *Pulse* writer believes doctors should discourage grown men from playing soccer and rugger in their later years. Nor should they condone middle-aged men donning running kit and sprinting away into the dawn.

'Dieting as a means of controlling body weight has the advantage,' he points out, 'that it may be pursued without detriment for the whole life of the person concerned and not just for a limited period.'

The point is valid in the context of this book, since the long-livers of Ecuador, the Caucasus and Hunza do, if largely from force of circumstance, diet the whole of their lives. Fat people are virtually unknown in their communities and, on the rare occasions when they appear, tend to excite only ridicule. Somehow, although there are occasions when centenarians, particularly in the USSR, take part in sprinting races, they do not train for them; it is all done on the spur of the moment – in the way that men may enter for the fathers' race at a school sports day in the West.

Exercise in the rural longevity areas is taken daily in the course of work in the fields; though unhurried it is consistent. Otherwise there is walking and horse-riding. Although the life of the super-centenarians must always be considered quantitatively, there is more than enough evidence that it has quality too. And the basis of this quality lies in their sincere religious beliefs, whether they be Roman Catholics (as is the case of the Ecuadorans), Mohammedans (Hunzukuts) or a mixture of Islamic and Russian Orthodox religions (the Caucasians).

Religion, of course, has played a fundamental part in the evolution of all mankind. Religion has organized peoples into separate communities, led to bloody conflict, introduced the notion of law and order, caused frightful sectarian crimes and brought peace beyond understanding. The worship of God, whether through Christian, Jewish or Muslim eyes, has always tended to be a family affair. Every consideration of 'going to church' evokes the picture of well-behaved families setting out together to church or synagogue to hear what the local preacher has to say. It is as true a picture today as it was in the Middle Ages.

And in this picture lies the notion of family unity even if at times, as in the Victorian era, it was achieved by severe if not actually cruel paternal strictures. Nowadays, in the Western world, the total family involvement in religion is less in evidence but Dr Davies in his illuminating book, *The Centenarians of the Andes* (Barrie & Jenkins), shows that this age-old custom is still as strong as ever among the villagers.

The Vilcabambans are not, it seems, troubled by religious doubts but retain an implicit belief in Almighty God and his good intentions for them. The Roman Catholic religion, Dr Davies says, was introduced to the Andean Indians by Catholic missionaries following in the wake of the Conquistadores. It is thought, by the way, that the name Vilcabamba may have had its origin in the language of the Quechua Indians and should be translated as 'Sacred Valley', although this is not the only possibility. Local legend also has it that the valley was the original paradise from which Adam and Eve were cast out. In support of this admittedly suspect notion, Dr Davies writes:

There are no harmful reptiles there . . . neither we nor anyone we met has ever seen any. Nor are there giant harmful insects, spiders, centipedes or dangerous mosquitoes, or harmful animals.

All this adds to the legend that the area is a paradise with special and sacred sites. The sacredness of these sites goes back to pre-Colombian times – that is, to the time of the Incas and, who knows, perhaps even before. There are no written histories. All around these villages are signs of prehistoric activities, old village sites, the stones of hut circles and marks on the mountainsides of cultivated fields from days gone by, which are much less rarely found near villages in other areas of southern Ecuador.

It is, of course, from the carefully kept records of long-dead Catholic priests that Dr Davies was able to confirm to his own satisfaction the great ages of people he met on several visits to Vilcabamba and other areas of longevity. It hardly seems that any priest would have been party to exaggeration in this respect; he would not have given a thought to the notion that anyone in future years would be remotely interested in the ages of his parishioners.

Dr Davies says the beautiful church of Vilcabamba was built 150 years ago on the site of other churches dating back centuries earlier. On Sundays the church is the focal point for people coming in from a wide surrounding area for midday mass.

Unfortunately the task of checking the precise ages of the Russians and Hunzukuts is not as simple and, in fact, cannot be done through religious documents. Reliance has to be placed on military records, inter-state passports and even hearsay. But the same kind of deep religious convictions seem to uphold the people of Hunza and the Caucasus. All references to Shirali Muslimov, for example, emphasize the fact that he said his prayers every day at sunrise; and it is reasonable to suppose that this example would have been followed by the majority of his large family.

In general, the prerequisites of a long and healthy life are not difficult to appreciate and apply everywhere in the world, whether or not people actually reach the age of a hundred or more. Dr Davies comments, 'If we take an overall look at England we find that those people who are working in agriculture live the longest, followed closely by clergymen; then come amateur naturalists. These groups also have the lowest incidence of cancer. Most are thought to have a capacity to relax; they are also less surrounded by polluted air. Also, at least until recently, these three groups were not noted for their wealth and could not afford rich food – plain food was the order of the day.'

10 Death is unnatural

As humanity enters the last quarter of the twentieth century one thing is predominantly apparent. We are, for the first time in our long and strange history, coming to terms with the Universe around us. Of course, it is only a start and a rather tentative one at that.

But the fact remains that our spaceships have taken men to the moon and back. Others, unmanned, have given us close-up pictures of some of the planets in our solar system including Venus, Mars and Jupiter. There is also a spacecraft going to Saturn. But, more than this, another one is on its way to the very boundary of the solar system; and the time will come when it quits the solar system altogether and heads out for the distant stars carrying with it Mankind's first message to any other intelligent creatures it might encounter in the limitless depths of space.

But, as things are, since the travelling distance and time required for the journey are so vast, the chances of anybody on earth today being still alive to receive a reply – should it ever come – are inconceivably remote. Nor is it likely that our descendants many generations from now will be alive to receive the message even though, technologically, they will probably be in a better position to do so.

Only in the case of space missions accomplished very close

to the earth can today's scientists hope to remain alive long enough to see the completion of their work. That is indeed the grumble of so many people besides scientists in this modern age: that life is too short to do the things they want to do and, in many cases, must do.

Death, it can be argued, is against human nature. Man has always felt, albeit subconsciously, that the aeons spent in the process of his evolution are wasted if, in the end, he is allotted little more than seventy years of earthly life. That is probably why Man has always had visions of eternal life and why every religion or faith has always promised him immortality if only in 'heaven'.

According to many of the world's gerontologists, death is an unnatural process and it is becoming evident that Man must devise a much longer active life on earth before he can undertake any long space journey.

Yet death, oddly enough, has had an important part to play in life, making possible the appearance and retention by natural selection of forms of life best adapted to their environment. Without death, in fact, our animal forebears would never have evolved into men. But in this process death established, not only for us but for all living species, a 'natural' span of life. We are directly descended from primates whose life-span was limited to approximately the time needed to leave a viable posterity behind, thus ensuring the survival of the species. Why otherwise should our basic and predominant instincts be those of survival and self-preservation? Why otherwise should we have endeavoured throughout the centuries to discover or devise a means of living longer and retaining our youthful vitality?

On becoming a social creature, Man opted out of natural

selection. Thus the late Vasily Kuprevich, president of the Byelorussian Academy of Sciences and a vigorous opponent of the notion that death is inevitable, once wrote: 'For Man death has become an historical anachronism. From the standpoint of society it is harmful. In the light of the problems facing humanity it is absurd. And who wants to perpetuate absurdity for all time?'

Some people believe that there is a pre-ordained, God-given upper limit of, say, eighty to a hundred years to human life. But nobody really knows the greatest age to which man has ever lived. Some gerontologists think that 120 years is the limit. But, as we have seen, others are prepared to accept the claims of people who say they are 150 years old or more. There is, in fact, no way of proving scientifically that ageing and death are inevitable. It is really a notion which Man has conditioned himself to accept.

Pavlov's dogs, put into situations in which they were temperamentally unable to cope, perished before their time. This suggests that the processes of ageing and death are somehow linked to the nervous system; in other words, because the nervous system wears out. To quote Kuprevich again: 'The most important symptom of old age is progressive reduction in the regulation of the vital processes and a decline in their intensity.

'I believe that in the not-too-distant future the study of human mental activity will be built anew on new foundations, and that we shall find new psychotherapeutic ways and means of protecting the nervous system against wear and tear, and of regenerating it.'

From the foregoing it is apparent that the fight for longevity is basically concerned with what might be called programmed death. The theory advanced to account for programmed death is that billions of cells making up our bodies have an inbuilt mechanism enabling them to divide (and thus multiply to cause growth) only a limited number of times.

When that number comes up, so to speak, the body reaches its limit of development and comes to a halt. After that the cells only die and the body shrinks and weakens, eventually dying generally as well as locally.

If this theory is correct, scientists face the not inconsiderable task of finding out how the death programme can be altered and cells encouraged to go on dividing indefinitely in a regular and healthy manner. The theory implies, of course, that heredity must play a part in determining the length of our lives although this may differ slightly from individual to individual.

On the other hand, it may be that the body somehow accumulates deleterious materials in its tissues to such an extent that the cells become unable to perform their normal functions efficiently. But it is more than likely that no single process is responsible for ageing and that other factors including environmental influences contribute to slowing down, shrinking and dying.

Experiments have shown that rats kept in a cold laboratory outlive those kept in a warm one – presumably because their metabolism is slowed down. It has also been observed that underfed rats live longer than well-fed ones. Even the amount of sunlight a living being receives may play a part, for the cells of certain plants die more quickly if the plants are exposed to light for a long time. Metabolism is again increased.

The late Dr Alexis Carrel of the Rockefeller Institute for Medical Research is reported to have kept a heart taken from a chicken embryo beating and growing in a culture dish for more than twenty-five years. The heart in its natural environment of the chicken's body grows old and the bird dies from natural causes (if allowed to) in a few years. But the very unnatural environment of the laboratory meant that the heart cells were able to live on and on. All of which seems to contradict the notion of a programmed death. It is this sort of complexity and contradiction which constantly faces biologists studying the mysteries of ageing.

In recent times, there have been a number of scientifically backed theories on the ageing process. It seems that Nikita Mankovsky's vitality booster of polyvitamins, enzymes, microelements and amino acids is the most reasoned and rational of all. Indeed, when small amounts of these essential food factors are taken daily on an empty stomach, first thing in the morning, the results can be observed within a few weeks. Combined with occasional sweat baths and the avoidance of *animal* fats, they can undoubtedly revitalize the elderly and, if regular daily exercise is taken as well, it is no exaggeration to say that a rejuvenation is effected in a matter of months.

*

Quite the most eerie of theories about the ageing process is one put forward alleging the gradual failure of the human body to recognize itself. According to this theory, body tissues may undergo mutations through the years. They can then be attacked by the body's own defence mechanisms, involving antibodies which treat them as foreign tissue. The same antibodies which fight disease and enable us to recover our health might, it is suggested, mistake the body's own cells for foreign bodies and attack or destroy them. Trans-

91

plant surgery has dramatically emphasized how antibodies can cause the rejection of foreign tissue, and some scientists believe that this somewhat unlikely self-destruction could take place in old age.

Yet another theory suggests that ageing may be caused by a virus, though this is the least likely possibility. All these theories are mentioned mainly to show the enormous amount of work which has already been done and the wide range of researches which have been carried out on the ageing process.

The theory in this book, however, is that the body's failure to renew cells and tissues is at the root of the trouble and that essential food factors, including polyvitamins, enzymes, microelements and amino acids, if administered correctly, will stimulate the rebuilding and replacement of these. Since these factors become scarcer as we grow older, this seems to be a reasonable explanation of ageing. And, in fact, when these essential food factors are taken, the restoration of youthful vitality appears to take place very quickly. Many gerontologists and scientists support this view, though the problem of finding a low cost source of all these factors has long prevented their widespread use.

*

Since the tissues of our bodies are continually being renewed, it seems reasonable to suppose that continued life and vitality depend on this process of renewal. If we can find a suitable material which provides all these vital factors, then the problem of ageing in good health may at last have been solved.

From this brief survey of the puzzles which have cropped up in ageing research it appears that we have a long way to go before the whole mystery is solved. But, as in the case of many other medical problems, it is not necessary to know the facts before taking remedial action. Thus, for example, diabetes can be treated and the victims of this disease enabled to lead relatively normal lives although, in fact, they have not been cured.

Similarly, the elderly can attain youthful vitality again, though, of course, nothing will alter the fact that they were born before the Second World War.

Before concluding this chapter we must emphasize that, whatever theories may be advanced about ageing, there is a great deal we can do to prevent ourselves growing too old too soon. This has been admirably illustrated by Dr John Maddison of Twickenham, Middlesex, who has benefited hundreds of elderly people in the district – and elsewhere – by giving them similar preparations to those originally recommended by Nikita Mankovsky. Containing polyvitamins and minerals, Dr Maddison's treatment is based on the fact that his administration of essential food factors stimulates body cells and delays the onset of deterioration which usually begins in the mid-fifties.

This treatment might well be described as a food supplement, insofar as it also stimulates the glands. Women are reported to gain firmer, neater figures and men have a new spring in their step and a return of confidence. This is probably the first time a medical man in Britain has realized the importance of counteracting the initial stages of ageing by the administration of essential food factors. It is to be hoped, indeed, that many more doctors will follow the example of Dr Maddison, since the restoration of youthful vitality is not normally attempted by our medical profession.

11 Beware a fat bank account

The myths about ageing are many, but the list can be shortened to a basic ten. So let us take each of these ten in turn and see what can be said about their validity . . .

1 Man cannot add significantly to his life-span
Even without further research we can already find methods of increasing our life-span by fifteen to thirty years. Dietary control and a special regimen based on the lives of inhabitants of the 'regions of longevity' can make a profound difference. And animal experiments have shown that restricting diet to basic necessities-plus-roughage has a major effect upon life-span.

2 Greater longevity in good health can be achieved . . . but not in the near future
Besides the dietary restrictions mentioned above there is the possibility of living longer with the help of certain drugs and food additives or supplements.

3 Delaying the onset of old age and death will impose great economic burdens on society as a whole
The increase of long life cannot in general be achieved without improving the health of old people. In good health they can look after themselves to a greater extent and can remain

at work thereby, becoming a positive economic benefit. Just imagine how valuable would be the knowledge and experience of our great surgeons, musicians, architects, scientists and many others whose work may otherwise be cut short by death.

4 *Prolonging life for more and more people will give rise to new social problems, particularly between the old and the young*
Older people remaining in good health will 'think younger', and learn to see possible problems arising. They will know how to deal with them, and their experience and knowledge can be very useful to the younger members of their society. This has actually happened in Soviet states and in South America.

5 *Any increase in life-span would severely affect the population explosion*
Efforts to curb the population explosion are already beginning to have an effect, especially in the Western world, while Japan has recently reduced its average annual population growth-rate from 2.5 per cent to less than 1 per cent. Most Communist countries are already less than 1 per cent.

Furthermore, it has been estimated that if we could make the most of the world's resources, the earth could support twice its present population.

6 *We ought not to tinker with ageing because to do so is interfering with Nature*
We do not know enough yet about the problems to make any such sweeping assumption. But surely Nature must be in favour of continued survival and renewed vitality. What can be the harm in such a project? If we are to believe our own Bible, Methuselah was surely an example.

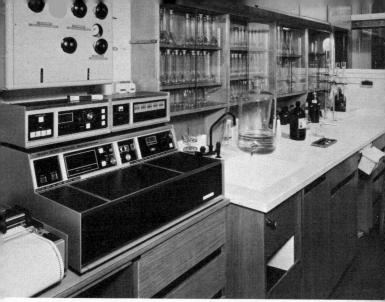

Above A corner of one of the laboratories where Pollen-B is converted into tablet form.

Below Sampling a delivery of bee-collected pollen, a substantial tonnage of which is imported annually.

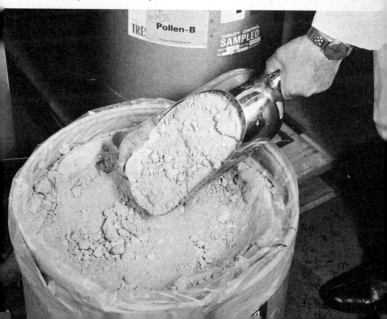

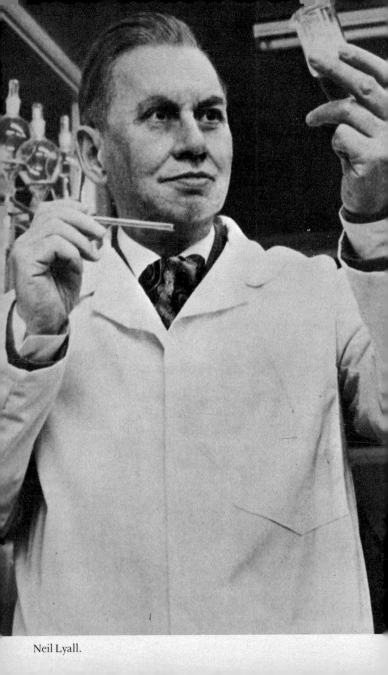

Neil Lyall.

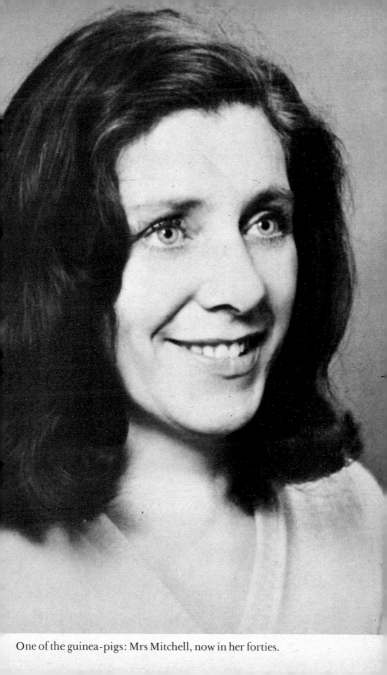

One of the guinea-pigs: Mrs Mitchell, now in her forties.

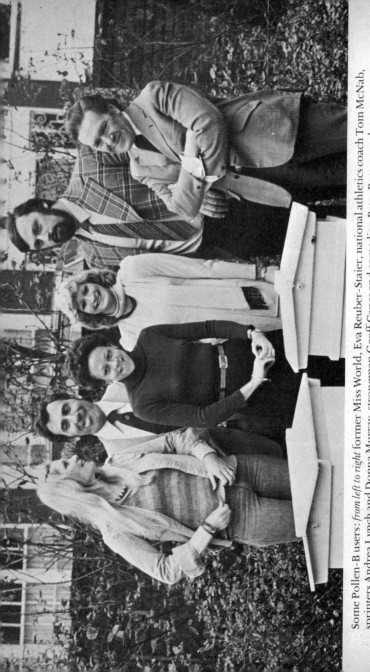

Some Pollen-B users: *from left to right* former Miss World, Eva Reuber-Staier, national athletics coach Tom McNab, sprinters Andrea Lynch and Donna Murray, strongman Geoff Capes and comedian Peter Butterworth.

7 The death of the elderly makes way for new, and possibly better people

This is the most presumptuous of all suggestions. Anyway, old people who have been revitalised can do more to help themselves and are unlikely to get in anyone's way. They could also help in the better development of the young.

8 Increasing the life-span could only lead to more and more decrepit people

We seem to have dealt with this before.

9 The present progress in the problems of ageing is all that can be expected

You must be joking. Not nearly enough research is going on. We have only scraped the surface. Who knows whether Man may not yet become able to live three hundred years?

10 Man has the potential to become physically immortal

Nature seems to have placed a limit on the duration of human existence. But the human mind has broken through many of Nature's limits. We have already visited the moon and we can travel faster than sound. We have already seen the benefits obtained by administration of polyvitamins, enzymes, micro-elements and amino acids – as established by one of the world's greatest gerontologists – Nikita Mankovsky.

And it appears that adjustments in our diet or consuming the right kind of food in the right quantities is what basically matters in keeping us fit and able to survive the vicissitudes of life and therefore to live a longer and more active life.

So now let us consider diet. But we must think of diet in its real sense, not merely as a means of slimming – the sort of activity that pretty young women engage in during the spring to ensure that they look their best in bikinis on summer holiday beaches. Diet is a serious matter which should concern us all our lives, not just when the fancy takes us. It should particularly concern us in our later years, when we are not as active as we used to be.

Mention the word 'diet' to most people and you soon become involved in an odd kind of arithmetic concerning calories. Everyone knows about calories – or do they? Look in a dictionary and you will find that a calorie is a 'unit of heat required to raise the temperature of one gramme of water through one degree Centigrade'. To very few people is this a meaningful definition and you may ask, 'What has it got to do with food anyway?'

The fact is that heat is a form of energy and we need energy to accomplish our daily tasks, so we obtain heat energy by chemically 'burning' food in our bodies. Foodstuffs vary. Some foodstuffs provide a lot of calories, others very few. What is necessary, therefore, is to ensure that our calorie intake is neither too high nor too low, according to what we do in the form of work and exercise to expend the calories we require. It is rather like a bank account. The calories paid in must be balanced by the calories paid out. Otherwise the bank account builds up and we get fat. Or the account becomes overdrawn and we become thin and weak through lack of energy.

When we are young and vigorous and always active, it doesn't matter so much if we eat a lot, and perhaps unwisely, because we are constantly putting our calories to energetic use in growing, in deliberate physical exercise and in general knocking about. But, in later years, especially after the age of fifty, we tend to slow down. We become less interested in exerting ourselves (a little gentle gardening will do) and we sit around more. But we still enjoy our food and, perhaps because we are sitting around, we eat even more. Thus because expenditure is slackening the calorie bank balance starts to build up to formidable proportions. Having no outlet, unused calories lodge, so to speak, all over our tissues, slowing us down still more in body and mind. Perhaps we become despondent and disappointed in ourselves and our accomplishments, or lack of them, and seek solace in absorbing even more calories.

This is when the obvious signs of ageing begin to appear. Clearly, there is a remedy – to reduce calorie intake and, if possible, take more exercise, even *some* exercise every day.

The important thing for people getting on in years is to recognize what foodstuffs are high in calories and cut down on them even if they cannot give them up altogether. Between the ages of twenty and forty, men who do not exert themselves require from 2,500 to 3,000 calories a day. Between forty and sixty the requirement drops to between 2,300 and 2,500. After sixty-five most can get by with a total of less than 2,300 although, of course, it depends on one's character, build and personality. Women require between three and five hundred calories a day less than men. Some people, as we have seen, remain active all their lives while others are only too ready to accept increasing age as an excuse to put their feet up. These are the ones most likely to become fat, eat more and grow older more quickly. It has been said that growing fat is tantamount to growing old and there is a strong basis of truth in this, since obesity is associated with atherosclerosis, the 'furring up' of arteries, consequent high blood-pressure and heart disease.

But let us examine, in terms of actual foodstuffs, what calorie intake is adequate for remaining vigorous and active as we grow older. Here are the basic items for a simple daily menu – with calorie values:

Breakfast

	calories
unsweetened fruit juice	5
cornflakes with bran	50
1 slice toast (wholemeal bread) with margarine	100
grilled kipper or 2 very thin rashers lean bacon	100
1 cup tea (without sugar)	5
breakfast total	260

Elevenses

1 cup tea, coffee	5

Lunch

consommé or clear soup	20
lean meat, green vegetables peas or beans	100
1 cup tea or coffee	5
elevenses and lunch total	130

Afternoon tea

1 wholemeal cake or biscuit	100
1 cup tea without sugar	5

Supper/dinner

consommé or clear soup	20
lean meat and green salad with extra vegetables	150
sweet (fruit or trifle – without cream)	75
tea and supper total	350

A cup of hot milk or cocoa may be taken on retiring for the night. The day's total calories only amount to about 750. This allows for an extra biscuit or an occasional cake when you feel hungry. The daily calorie intake does not exceed 1,000 and conforms to the sparse eating habits of the very old people living in regions of longevity. This diet may be increased so that 1,500 to 2,000 calories are consumed daily as a maximum. But the occasional glass of whisky on retiring or occasional sweets increase the calorie intake. This is not, of course, intended to be a rigid or invariable diet but the minimum required by the very old in order to maintain good health. It allows for the occasional nibble between meals which is almost unavoidable and forms a useful basis which can be varied. For example, extra green vegetables may be eaten according to one's appetite.

Chicken or fish may be eaten instead of lean meat and a half-teaspoonful of sugar taken to make tea or coffee more palatable. But the elderly do not normally require substantial meals and over-eating must always be avoided. Don't forget that the occasional alcoholic drink adds substantially to calorie intake.

After the age of sixty-five a maximum intake of 2,000 calories daily during the summer months and 2,500 daily in winter should be the limit. Generally speaking, we in Britain eat far too much. The long-livers of the world all eat sparsely and this seems to be one of the secrets of their vitality.

Heavy meals should be avoided. And sauces, condiments and relishes should be kept to a minimum. Simple, plain food at all times is the golden rule and a good supply of fresh vegetables and fruit will stave off any hunger which may occur between meals.

Since heavy work is seldom undertaken by the elderly there is no purpose in over-eating and it can be harmful. It is also prudent to select a diet which is low in cholesterol-producing foods. Note that animal fats including butter and lard should be avoided whenever possible and that certain vegetable oils actually tend to reduce cholesterol levels in the blood. The beneficial vegetable oils include maize or corn oil and soya bean oil. Margarine made from these oils is believed to be safer than butter. But we still have to consider these highly important substances known as essential food factors. These are the enzymes, vitamins and mineral salts or micro-elements and all of them are required in small amounts by the human body.

12 'Limeys' at sea

Vitamins are organic substances that the body cannot make for itself; they have to be obtained from what we eat. And without them we are soon in trouble, for vitamins (a term introduced by the Polish biochemist Casimir Funk in 1912) are most conspicuous by their absence.

Take the case of Vitamin C which, more than any other, has a place in history. It was Vitamin C (or ascorbic acid) that indirectly earned British seamen the name of 'limeys' and enabled them to dominate the trade routes of the world. The story goes back to the middle of the fifteenth century when long sea voyages first began to be made to obtain pepper and other spices from the East to relieve the dullness of European food, especially in winter when supplies of fresh food dwindled. Many sailors died from the effects of a disease called scurvy which caused bleeding from the gums, swelling of joints, general bruising of the body and, in advanced cases, fatal internal haemorrhage.

Scurvy invariably attacked crews at sea for long periods, whether the venture was for trade, exploration or war. Often, indeed, it made the difference between success and failure, and about three hundred years passed before anyone discovered that the disease could be prevented by including citrus fruits, especially limes, in the crews' diet. Probably the first long voyage when men did not develop scurvy was that made by Captain Cook and his men, when they discovered Australia in the 1770s.

The name 'limeys' was bestowed on British sailors by the Americans. Nobody knew then that their health was being maintained by ascorbic acid but in fact Vitamin C led to the growth and strength of the British Navy, which at last could stay at sea for months on end. Nowadays, of course, scurvy is a relatively rare disease. We obtain our Vitamin C not only from citrus fruits but also from fresh green vegetables.

When vitamins were first discovered they were all identified by letters of the alphabet, and these are still in use, but it is becoming increasingly common to employ their chemical names. Thus:

Vitamin A1	Retinol
Vitamin B1	Thiamine
Vitamin B2	Riboflavine
Vitamin B12	Cyanocobalamin
Vitamin C	Ascorbic acid
Vitamin D3	Cholecalciferol

The importance of Vitamin C has been briefly dealt with, so let us now consider the others in this short list and see what benefit they are to our health:

RETINOL This vitamin, as its name implies, is associated with vision. It assists us to see in a dim light and a deficiency of it leads to night-blindness, common in tropical Africa, parts of South-east Asia and the Middle East. It is not a serious condition in itself but should be regarded as a warning of more dangerous possible consequences.

Retinol is found only in foods of animal origin, especially liver; the livers of fish are a particularly rich source, hence the popularity of cod-liver oil for children. But Vitamin A can also be obtained from milk, butter, cheese and eggs.

THIAMINE Lack of sufficient thiamine in the body has long been known to be the cause of the disease called beriberi among the people of the East but in the last half-century the disease has steadily declined. It occurs either as a wasting disease (dry beriberi) or a swelling disease (wet beriberi), in which the body becomes waterlogged. An injection of the vitamin can have a dramatic effect, leading to recovery in a few hours. The lives of all animals and plants depend on thiamine, which assists body cells to make use of carbo-hydrates. The richest natural source of it is probably yeast, and foodstuffs which tend to be a poor source are mostly those which have been refined, including rice, certain flour and sugars. In some countries where a lot of bread made from finely milled wheat is eaten, there is a legal requirement to add thiamine.

RIBOFLAVINE If we are deprived of this vitamin we tend to get sores at the corner of the mouth or swollen and chapped lips. The tongue may become swollen and painful as well and the eyes develop a congested appearance especially round the cornea. Such conditions are common in parts of the world where people are afflicted with malnutrition. Both children and adults may show evidence of riboflavine deficiency but the condition is less serious than others; and may be seen in Britain and America, especially among the elderly, as well as in poorer countries.

Meat, eggs and fish are good sources of riboflavine. Useful

amounts can also be obtained from wheat; and beer drinkers will be pleased to learn that they can obtain a regular supply from their particular tipple.

CYANOCOBALAMIN This is a substance containing cobalt needed to safeguard us from what used to be called pernicious anaemia. Not a lot is known about it – except that it works and that as little as a millionth of a gramme a day may be enough to keep a patient in good health. Cyanocobalamin is available in small amounts in all animal tissues but the only rich source is the liver.

CHOLECALCIFEROL This vitamin plays an essential role in the strengthening of bones. A child lacking this vitamin may grow with soft bones which become twisted and deformed – a disease known as rickets. It used to be common throughout the world especially in the industrial cities of Europe at the end of the nineteenth century but thanks to proper preventative measures rickets is now a relatively minor medical problem. Again cod-liver oil is a rich source of this vitamin along with halibut oil and swordfish oil. But eggs and butter also contain appreciable amounts, and so does milk.

*

These, of course, are not the only vitamins needed to maintain a healthy body but they are among the most important. Without them, indeed, it would be impossible to lead a vigorous life; without some of them it would be impossible to live at all for very long. But even vitamins do not bring us to the end of the story. So complex are our bodies that we also have need for microscopic quantities of certain metallic elements as well – usually referred to as 'trace elements'. Some of them, like iron, for example, calcium, copper, magnesium and zinc we are accustomed to consider in very large quantities for industrial purposes; and it is surprising to learn that they play a part in keeping us alive and active. After all, iron is used for making locomotives, copper is put on the roofs of churches or made into steam boilers; zinc is sold in sheets for a variety of laboratory purposes, etc. But let us see what invisible amounts of these elements do for *us*.

CALCIUM We need calcium to build strong skeletons. The bones of the skeleton have usually grown to their maximum by the time we reach the age of twenty. During the next five years or so the bones thicken, but thereafter the tendency is for them to become thinner and more fragile until in our final years we risk a fracture from the slightest fall. But, in fact, bones once formed do not stay put all our lives. Bone material is continually being renewed with the help of calcium, though some of it is lost and excreted in urine. The precise mechanics of this turnover is not fully understood but we know it happens and, as mentioned earlier, we know that cholecalciferol (Vitamin D) plays an essential part in the process.

Fortunately, calcium is obtainable from all natural foods, animal or vegetable. But what we have to remember is that processed foods may contain none at all.

IRON Iron helps the blood transport oxygen to the brain. The red corpuscles derive their bright colour from this element. Without sufficient iron, indeed, they become paler. So, as a consequence, do we ourselves; we become anaemic and have a feeling of lassitude sometimes ascribed to 'tired blood' – one remedy for which is to take booster tablets containing iron.

Iron, like calcium, is not in short supply. It is present in

107

cereals and vegetables but we get about 30 per cent of our requirement from meat, and possibly 20 per cent from fish. Our iron balance, however, is fairly easily maintained because losses are small and mostly associated with the excretion of faeces and urine.

ZINC The failure of young people to grow to normal size and develop sexually has been noticed in areas where diet is deficient in this element. Zinc is believed to encourage chemical reactions in the body concerned with the absorption of proteins and carbohydrates. Foodstuffs derived from animals are good sources of this element, especially beef, pork, lamb, fish and other seafoods.

MAGNESIUM Although we have a surprisingly large amount of this element in our bodies – perhaps as much as twenty-five grammes – its importance has been realized only comparatively recently. Magnesium appears to be needed for a great many chemical processes, particularly those concerned with oxydization. Without sufficient magnesium we are likely to develop acute diarrhoea, kidney failure and malnutrition and, if we are not careful, become chronic alcoholics. We also tend to become irritable and emotionally unstable – which is hardly surprising. But fortunately magnesium, again, is plentiful in both vegetables of all sorts and meat, especially viscera. Milk, on the other hand, is a poor source of magnesium.

COPPER Like magnesium, copper is also believed to have an important role in oxydization processes in the body, and to facilitate the synthesis of iron into haemoglobin; but the precise mechanism is another biochemical mystery. Older people rarely if ever suffer from copper deficiency, but some children do and become anaemic as a result. The richest sources of dietary copper include kidney, liver, shellfish, nuts and raisins.

FLUORINE is another element of which we should take account, particularly in view of its affinity for bones and teeth. Fluorine indeed is considered an essential nutrient in providing resistance to dental caries and decay. The fluoridation of water supplies, though strongly opposed from some quarters, is regarded by the World Health Organization as 'a highly important public health measure' in areas where natural water supplies do not contain a sufficient concentration of fluoride.

Before leaving the subject of trace elements perhaps it should be mentioned that the list of those which benefit the body includes CHROMIUM, COBALT, MOLYBDENUM and SELENIUM. One could be pardoned for thinking indeed that with so much needed to ensure that we remain in constant good health, it is surprising that we manage to live so long, let alone feel able to contemplate increasing our life-span.

13 Last and best years

Are you looking forward to a cosy, well-earned retirement or does the prospect of living on a pension, even what is sometimes called a 'top hat' pension, fill you with gloom? Such questions deserve consideration because doctors are tending to accept the notion that it is just not good enough to put people 'out to grass' simply because they have reached retirement age – whatever that may be.

Some ought to go earlier, they say, and some ought to be allowed to stay at work as long as they feel fit enough and wish to continue. Some men, for example, feel it is ridiculous to give up their jobs at a sprightly age of sixty-five while others are ready to put their feet up in their mid fifties. The point was firmly made at a World Health Organization conference meeting in 1974 by Dr Georges Lambert, head of France's occupational health services.

Dr Lambert called for a new understanding of what retirement was all about. Instead of slavishly persisting with chronological retirement, he said, we should start thinking in terms of biological retirement. Family doctors, playing a much greater part than they do today, should be called upon to make individual assessments of old people, case by case, and their retirement advice should be based on the personal capabilities and wellbeing of those concerned.

Doctors should know their patients' life-styles to the extent that they could not only recognize someone with many good working years left in him but could also detect signs of premature ageing and try to do something about them.

It does not matter, of course, if a man (or woman) approaching retirement has something to look forward to. He or she may have planned a completely new career and be only too anxious to get on with it. The trouble and the tragedy comes when there is nothing to look forward to and when the future looms up in hopeless blankness.

Having something to anticipate, be it no more than a birthday party, may have a greater effect on our wellbeing than is generally realized, an American sociologist once postulated. Pleasurable anticipation of a future event might actually help to prolong life, reported David Phillips of Johns Hopkins University after making a study of elderly people.

Mr Phillips began by checking 1,251 Americans listed as people who had achieved distinction in their lifetime. Very few, he found, had died just before their birthdays, whereas a large number had died during a period of three months afterwards. Was this significant?

To check further, Mr Phillips turned to the records of Jewish communities in New York and Budapest. In both cases he found a marked decline in the death rate during the month before Yom Kippur, the Jewish Day of Atonement. And records show a similar decline, he reported, before every American election from 1904 to 1964 when the population could be assumed to be more than usually interested in the future.

The logic of looking forward is obvious. It implies not only faith in the future but curiosity to see what happens next and curiosity has been a motivating factor for humanity throughout the ages.

American psychologists are now considering the possibility that men and women condition themselves to an inevitable process of ageing. Brought up to accept religious beliefs that the life span of mankind is threescore years and ten they kid themselves that they must begin to slow down a bit after the age of fifty. Next, they begin to enjoy the little courtesies which are generally accorded to the elderly and the deference accorded them by younger people. They like having things done for them. And they soon become demanding in their requests. Many elderly people resolutely refrain from carrying heavy articles; they begin to expect people to stand aside and give way to them on account of their age and ask others to fetch and carry all manner of things for them which they could quite easily manage for themselves.

This psychological self-conditioning can make many old people a burden to relatives and friends. And their eventual dependence on others can become quite a social problem. By the time such people are sixty they can tend to become intolerable and their later years are filled with boredom.

Of course, adapting to age is largely a personal matter. The elderly often have to create their own interests by starting a new career, taking up a new hobby or adopting an entirely new life-style. What we must all beware of is 'thinking old'. When circumstances oblige us to withdraw from normal work it is all too easy to condition ourselves, albeit subconsciously, into feeling that we are 'past it'. The man who buys himself a walking-stick may soon come to believe that he really needs the thing . . . to depend on it until it becomes a crutch. Already he is beginning to think of himself as an old man and, pretty soon, others will think of him as an old man, too.

He may cling to a hearing-aid that for most of the time he could well do without. He may also adopt old-fashioned dressing habits. It all goes towards making him really old.

Similarly, there is the woman who decides that she should no longer wear a pretty coloured hat or dress but something more sedate. Soon she finds herself expecting a younger person to give up a seat for her in a bus or to help her across the road. It is very pleasant to command attention, of course, but as soon as she begins to think of it as her right she is on her way to being old and soon feels quite genuinely that she can no longer do things for herself.

She will be constantly popping a peppermint into her mouth to 'revive' herself or sniffing delicately at a lace handkerchief.

When all this starts, nobody can tell, but the prudent person will be on guard and do anything possible to retain independence and respect. What must be remembered is that retired people – generally from sixty onwards, let us say – may have as many years left to live as they had of working life . . . even without trying.

A great deal has been written about preparation for retirement both by doctors and laymen. It is not difficult to obtain information and advice not only on keeping happily occupied but on maintaining health, taking exercise, the use of medicine, how to cope with financial problems.

Elderly people cannot expect to retain full physical strength, and the gradual failure of eyesight and hearing can be vexing problems; but one thing the elderly can always take pride in is their continuing ability to make sound judgements. Nor is there any reason, whatever bludgeonings of fate they may have to endure, why they should lose their sense of humour.

If you are old and alone it is very easy to become self-centred and retreat from community life. So it is important to exercise self-discipline and make a point of joining in local affairs – even to the extent of eventually running them. There are clubs to which you can belong, and most local authorities organize afternoon or evening classes for senior citizens to learn new skills – to become passable musicians or artists – or even makers of handicraft objects.

Many an 'old' man or woman has discovered a hidden talent in this way. Not a few have found romance and a new life altogether. A lot depends, of course, on one's temperament. But in the first place it is a matter of health, which means having regular and balanced meals and taking sufficient exercise. The human body, as we have seen, is basically an engine and like all engines its good functioning depends upon careful maintenance. This surely is the lesson to be learned from the old folk of the Caucasus, Ecuador and Hunza.

People growing old towards the end of the twentieth century have more in their favour than at any time in the history of the world. Perhaps we should not think in terms of retirement at all, because of its connotation with 'giving up'. Instead we should think of embarking on a new phase of life, with new and even exciting problems to solve.

Apart from what we can do for ourselves to keep fit, it is comforting to know that medical science is improving all the time. In a few years the dread of cancer may have faded into the past. Replacement surgery (no longer bedevilled by the rejection problem) will take care of damaged hearts, livers and kidneys. Research doctors may even find a way of providing sight for the blind and hearing for the deaf. Crippling diseases will be mastered and new drugs developed to improve intellectual capacity, reduce obesity and stimulate sexual potency well beyond the time at which it normally begins to flag.

Health education will undergo rapid expansion; and new ideas, probably involving new professions, will come into being. For more and more people, being a centenarian will no longer involve dependence on others and a sense of uselessness. The last years of life may also be the best years.

In his splendid booklet, *Sixty Plus*, published by the British Medical Association, Dr John Maddison put it thus:

> Those of us in retirement should have faith in ourselves. We have an important place in society because we have the experience of a lifetime to give those who care to discuss things with us.
>
> We must think of old age as a time of tranquillity and fulfilment, giving us a chance to take things more easily; for independence; for freedom to do new things. Then retirement will be anticipated with equanimity and joy.
>
> Many of us complain all our lives that we never have any spare time for leisure. We would dearly love to write, to paint, to join a singing group, to go to the theatre, to play golf, to ramble in the countryside, to travel and go to foreign countries, to read, to do jobs around the house, to attend classes ... if only there were time ...
>
> From retirement onwards ... there is time!

14 A search for the secret

Neil Lyall's interest in longevity had been greatly aroused by Dr Ana Aslan's treatment of patients attending her clinic at the Institute of Geriatrics in Bucharest. His inquiries, however, persuaded him that procaine therapy could have only a temporary effect on physical wellbeing. Old people taking the treatment might feel younger, they might even look younger but the treatment was not basic enough, certainly not natural enough to add significantly to the length of their lives.

From reports he had read there were, however, parts of the world where people took old age for granted – people who had no access to any form of rejuvenation treatment, however effective, and had probably never even heard of it.

The first thing, therefore, was to test the strength of such reports, to satisfy himself that people of the Caucasus, Hunza, Vilcabamba and neighbouring areas of Ecuador really did live to ages of 150 or more, as was claimed. It was not easy. To have done so to his complete satisfaction would have involved a great deal of time-consuming and expensive travel to places largely cut off from ordinary life.

But there were other sources of information, such as foreign embassies and medical institutes specializing in the problems of old age, from which reliable evidence ought to be available. In the early 1960s Lyall set himself the task of collecting scientific papers and reports to further his researches. It was tedious and sometimes exasperating work, but the more he pursued it the more Lyall became convinced that extreme longevity was a fact, that Shirali Muslimov, Shirin Gazanov, Miguel Carpio and the rest of them were actually as old as they were said to be.

What really would be the point in either they or anyone else pretending otherwise, especially in the face of the growing medical interest these people were beginning to arouse in the world? The thing to do was to look for some special factor shared by the long-livers enabling them to survive against odds which had clearly defeated their contemporaries in other parts of the world.

This indeed was what some authors of scientific articles had already attempted to do, tentatively ascribing the phenomenon of healthy, active extreme old age either to clear, unpolluted mountain air and/or the quality of local drinking water, containing perhaps vital minerals which got lost at lower altitudes. Lyall himself was at first attracted to the notion that clean mountain air and water played a significant part in promoting longevity.

This notion, however, suffered a severe blow when his inquiries took him to Norway with a fellow-scientist. In a report on the visit, Lyall wrote:

We had trekked inland from the port of Bergen, striking North towards the Jotunheimen, probably the highest region in Norway. Certainly the air and water were clean and pure. Pollution was unknown. We hitch-hiked from village to village and stayed at local hotels on our way.

We noticed that large cans of sardines remained open for days on dining-room tables and we were told that the air was so clean that food remained edible for much longer. Here, then, were what we believed to be the ideal conditions for longevity. There appeared to be plenty of salmon trout and other fish in the sparkling fjords or lakes, and lean meat was plentiful.

However, we noticed a shortage of green vegetables. The subsoil was only a few centimetres deep and beneath lay solid rock ... Nor were there many flowers in these mountainous regions. We spoke to many old-looking men and women but could find none who were more than about sixty years of age. Clearly, the mountains which stretched across into Sweden were by no means a bastion of longevity.

In pursuit of an explanation to the puzzle of longevity Lyall made other visits to mountainous areas relatively near at hand, particularly in the Ardennes of Southern Belgium. There he found vegetables and flowers growing in greater abundance, but there was no evidence that people lived beyond the normal span. Mountain air and water were clearly of secondary importance. It was much more likely, he decided, that something in the diet of the Caucasians and their fellow long-livers elsewhere in the world kept them going.

'To test this theory,' he wrote, 'I travelled to a mild and lush area in the North of Scotland – the Moray Firth. Banff-shire and Moray were the regions that interested me most. The beautiful valley of the Deveron and Cromdale Hills south of Elgin were especially interesting ... for there I found many active old men of eighty and ninety.

'For some reason this is one of the mildest regions of the British Isles, in spite of its being in the extreme north. The air is pure and pollution is minimal and the area is noted for its long, late summer during which it is possible to read a newspaper outdoors at 11 p.m., owing to the extended hours of daylight.'

It was in Moray that Lyall first noticed the presence of bees in abundance. There had been none in the mountains of Norway and relatively few in the Ardennes of Southern Belgium, but bee-keeping was a popular activity in the North of Scotland and local 'heather honey' had a significant part in the diet of the people.

Honey, he remembered, was well-known to be of dietary value. People had eaten it throughout the ages and some exaggerated claims had been made for it.

In view of this, the possibility that the activities of bees and bee-keepers might hold the secret of longevity did not quickly occur to him. Several months after the trip to Scotland he came across a paper by a leading Soviet biologist, Nicolai Tsitsin, on the centenarians of Azerbaydzhan. In this paper, Tsitsin had put forward the theory that the extreme old age and vitality of the mountain people, many of whom were bee-keepers, was due to their habit of eating bee-collected pollen which became mixed with honey which the bees dropped on the floor of hives on their return from foraging.

Pure honey from the hives was sold by the bee-keepers in the ordinary course of making a living, but the 'contaminated' honey scrap which they scraped out when cleaning their hives was kept and eaten by themselves. Was there something in bee-collected pollen that was lacking in pollen that was wind-blown from grass or fell from trees?

Pollen, of course, occurs abundantly in spring and summer throughout the world. It fills the air and can often be seen as a greenish film on the surface of lakes and ponds. Some of it, as hay-fever sufferers know only too well, can cause misery.

Eyes water and noses run; headaches and feverishness distress people who are allergic. That is why the Asthma Research Council takes aerial pollen counts daily in Britain, from early June to mid July, so that when the count is going to be high, victims of hay-fever can be given advance warning and advised to stay indoors. This pollen is almost entirely from grass, notably varieties called Timothy and Crowsfoot, which are blown into the air by the wind or 'churned up' by gardeners mowing their lawns at weekends. Just a few microscopic grains may be enough to start a severe hay-fever attack in a particularly sensitive person. But pollen is essential for the fertilization of plants of all kinds and must therefore possess powerful properties. It also varies enormously from one species of plant to another.

The thought gave Lyall a further line of research aimed at obtaining laboratory analyses of pollen of all kinds from all parts of the world. And it was while he was pursuing this objective that a second piece of the jigsaw fell into place.

Another scientific paper, this time from the Russian gerontologist, Nikita Mankovsky, came into his hands in response to a letter he had written to Moscow. The paper outlined the considered opinion of the gerontologist that amino acids, polyvitamins, microelements and enzymes were basically what was needed to counter the effects of ageing in the middle years and restore vitality to the elderly.

Amino acids are important constituents of proteins, which are the building blocks of living tissue. These, together with microelements (salts of common metals like iron, zinc, phosphorus, magnesium and copper), need constant replacement to keep the human body in good repair. Enzymes are less easy to identify, but play the role of catalysts in encouraging and stimulating amino acids and microelements to do their job properly.

Lyall, through contact with bee-keepers' associations abroad, had already satisfied himself that bee-keeping was popular with the people of Hunza and Vilcabamba and that these people also ate honey scrap that would contain pollen from flowers which the bees had fertilized and which was fine enough to cling to the hairs of their legs and drop off again when they returned with their loads of nectar.

What remained was to discover whether this bee-collected pollen was much the same in all regions of longevity and whether, as Tsitsin had suggested, it contained any substance of value in promoting and maintaining the health of human beings. Analysing pollen grains is a long and difficult business, not lightly undertaken by any laboratory. But in the course of his inquiries Lyall was able to obtain an analysis of bee-collected honey already carried out by the Lee Foundation for Nutritional Research, Milwaukee, USA.

To his delight he found that bee-collected pollen contained, albeit in minute amounts, all the factors specified by Mankovsky as contributing to vigorous old age. In fact, it appeared, this pollen contained no less than fourteen vitamins, eleven enzymes, eleven minerals or microelements and nineteen amino acids.*

The Lee Foundation analysis came as a revelation. All that Lyall had been able to discover about the ordinary diet of the long-livers suggested that it was pretty frugal, consisting basically of lean meat or fish, fresh vegetables and fruit. At the same time, although there were notable exceptions, many

*see appendix

of them were heavy smokers and drinkers – of their own wine and home-grown tobacco.

On the face of it there seemed no good reason why they should live any longer than people elsewhere, apart perhaps from the fact that they had little or no access to factory food in tins and packets which was low in nutritional value. But as they were constantly, if unconsciously, supplying themselves with the amino acids, microelements, vitamins and enzymes which generally tend to become scarce in the diets of other old people, this might well account for their long and vigorous lives; especially as good health would keep them energetic and happy to work out-of-doors for many hours a day.

It was at this point that Neil Lyall had an inspiration which was to keep him busy for the next eight years and cost him, he estimates, about £20,000. Suppose pollen of the same quality as that which bees collected from flowers in the Caucasus, Ecuador and Hunza could be obtained from regions nearer at hand? Suppose it could be collected in bulk and brought to England. Then perhaps the pollen could be processed and prepared in tablet form for the benefit of people, old and young, not only in the British Isles but on the Continent and even further afield.

Lyall had a vision of marketing a product which would correct endless minor ailments by the simple method of supplementing their diet in the same way that it was apparently being supplemented in distant Vilcabamba, Hunza and Azerbaydzhan. People who had never heard of Shirali Muslimov, Shirin Gazanov or José David might themselves be able to live well beyond a hundred years in excellent health.

*

Throughout the 1960s Lyall dedicated himself to checking the quality of pollen throughout the Western world. As a leading food scientist he knew all about honey and was in touch with bee-keeping associations. He wrote to many of them requesting samples of honey 'contaminated' by pollen. Samples sealed in polythene bags arrived at his home near Richmond, Surrey, at regular intervals, from Canada, the Balkan states, Scandinavia and France. But the quality of pollen from most sources was so poor that Lyall could reject it almost on sight. Once in a while, however, he received a sample sufficiently fine for him to refer it for examination to Thomas Lachlan, who for years had been a London public health analyst and who is now operating a laboratory in St John's Wood. Eventually, however, there came a day when Lyall received a sample from south-eastern Europe which was almost exactly what he had hoped for.

'I could hardly believe it,' he said. 'As soon as it came I knew it was what I had been looking for. I knew also that there was a great deal more to be obtained from the same area of southern Europe, a constant supply, indeed. All I had to do was to arrange for bulk supplies to be collected and delivered.'

It was not, however, as simple as that. First he had to be sure the pollen *was* bee-collected, a process that involved the capturing of bees in selected areas and the brushing off of pollen from their legs for further careful examination. The best areas, Lyall discovered, were in southern and south-east Europe, especially Hungary and southern France. He found that bees in these areas were collecting pollen from blossoms similar to those found in the areas of longevity. There were blossoms of apple, pear, plum, cherry, peach and apricot, and many varieties of wild and cultivated flowers which also grew in Ecuador, Hunza and the Caucasus.

After months of inquiries and visits to farming areas in southern and south-east Europe Lyall and a group of colleagues assisting with the project set up, with the help of bee-keepers' associations, an organization for collecting bee-pollen from nearly a thousand hives, over hundreds of square miles.

By early 1971, nearly two hundred people were being paid to visit the hives and collect pollen and take it to central collecting stations, where it was stored in 5-kg polythene bags and packed into special drums for transport to England.

The pollen was collected, and still is, from small traps like egg-cups fitted with tiny brushes (to sweep the bees' legs as they entered the hives) which had earlier been placed in position. These traps had been bought from a manufacturing firm in Sweden and distributed when the collecting organization was first established. When you realize that every beehive accommodates from forty thousand to fifty thousand bees it is not surprising that, though only very small amounts of pollen are brought back by each bee, the amount in the trap quickly grows, and in practice it is found desirable for collectors to visit the hives at least twice a week to empty the traps. Many tons of bee-collected pollen are held in stock in Britain; and, with Nature producing fresh supplies every season, there is unlikely to be a shortage in the foreseeable future.

Unfortunately, it is not worth collecting pollen from beehives in the British Isles, largely because we do not have sufficient sunshine to guarantee either the quality or quantity required. It would just not be an economic proposition. And, in any case, even at the best of times the climate is too humid, and the pollen season is not long enough.

Even after the first commercial quantities of pollen from south-eastern Europe arrived in Britain, the problem was far from solved. Great care had to be taken to prevent the pollen from deteriorating while it was being processed for making into tablets. In fact, quality control measures were introduced at every stage.

Lyall himself devised a gentle air-drying process that could be regulated to ensure that the delicate substances remained in prime condition throughout. It was, in fact, nearly five years before the whole organization, from collecting to tabletting and packaging, was fully established. Then began months of negotiations with the medicines committee of the Department of Health and the Ministry of Agriculture before the golden-yellow tablets were permitted to be used in trials with human volunteers, and finally began to appear on the home market under the brand name Pollen-B . . . a supplementary food.

This bee-collected pollen in tablet form is now available in chemists and health-food shops throughout Britain and in most countries of the Continent. Pollen-B is recommended for people of all ages; for the young to keep them 'toned up', especially if they use a lot of energy in sporting activities; for the middle-aged to counteract that end-of-day feeling and ensure a full and active life; and for the elderly to ensure they are not deprived of dietary factors which are essential to give them vigour and enthusiasm to live beyond the normal span.

Anyone who has difficulty in obtaining supplies of Pollen-B locally has only to contact the manufacturers, Wassen Developments, Walton-on-Thames, Surrey. On payment of whatever amount is required packets are dispatched post free.

15 The guinea-pigs

On holiday in Austria in 1974 Vincent B. climbed a high mountain – right up to the snow-line. It was not easy because the effort also involved keeping up with a party of much younger people.

But the point is that he *wanted* to make that journey and enjoyed every minute of it. And on returning to his Surrey home this middle-aged family man, assisted by a neighbour, cut down nineteen pine trees in the course of clearing the woodlands he owns. He wanted to do that, too, although the job, including chopping the trees into small logs, took three weeks.

For, at the age of fifty-five, Vincent felt young again, not only physically but mentally. Life, as he put it, had become a challenge. Yet only two years earlier Vincent had felt like giving up. Everything was 'getting on top of him', he complained.

He had no specific illness but he felt listless and became tired easily. The effort to establish a business and bring up a family had left him feeling – and looking – his age. The idea of climbing a mountain would never, in those early days, have entered his head and as for tackling nineteen tall pine trees ... you had to be joking!

Vincent B. was one of the first 'guinea-pigs' Neil Lyall

invited to test the pollen pills which, after fourteen years' research and development were being produced in limited quantities.

The two men had met and become friends through lunching at the same restaurant at Ham, near Richmond, Surrey. On hearing Vincent complain of always feeling fagged out, Lyall asked him to try taking a pollen pill every morning and another before going to bed to see if they did any good.

The result, says Vincent, was 'staggering'. Within three months he was already feeling a new man and after taking bee-collected pollen for a year it seemed that nothing could get him down. He really felt at least ten years younger!

Vincent B. runs a precision tool designing concern employing more than twenty skilled men, and the slightest mistake on his part could have serious consequences. 'The responsibility used to worry me,' he said, 'and I would crawl home in the evenings fit for nothing and fall asleep in front of the telly. But it doesn't happen any more. I am much more alert than I have been for ten years and I don't need half so much sleep. I work harder and walk more. I mow the lawns at the weekends and have a good time with my two kids.'

He added, 'I feel completely revitalized and I must put it down to taking Pollen-B because I have had no medical attention and I never swallow any other kind of pills . . . not even an aspirin.'

This particular guinea-pig has noticed something else, too. Although he formerly suffered from at least one very severe cold every winter, he has not had a single cold for the last three years. Nor lost a single day through any illness. The notion of living to an age of a hundred years or more no longer strikes him as unlikely. In fact, Vincent is determined to do so.

Another Pollen-B guinea-pig is Ronald S., manager of a TV and radio store, who is also middle-aged. When Lyall first encountered him he was in poor health and low spirits. Ron was feeling 'down in the mouth' and, like Vincent B., he had little to look forward to.

But today he is feeling, and looking, younger and brighter. Ron has lost three stone in weight and become noticeably more 'alive'. He said that he only needed a few hours' sleep and woke refreshed and ready to face the day whatever its problems although previously everything had tended to get him down. 'I take a Pollen-B pill every morning without fail,' he added. 'I am sure they help me to cope with everything.'

In some ways, Miss Rosamund C. is the most remarkable example. Miss C. was nearly seventy when Lyall suggested that she tried Pollen-B. All her adult life she had suffered from severe arthritis and in her later years she could scarcely walk for the pains in her back and knee-joints.

Within a few months of taking bee-collected pollen she had regained a remarkable degree of relief and independence. The back pains had etched lines of suffering on her face and these have been smoothed away – like the pains in her back. She still has to walk slowly, often with the aid of a stick but she manages to cross a busy main road to her favourite coffee house and back again. Eventually she expects that her knee-joints will also benefit, but she is already able to get about and enjoy life considerably more than previously.

Lyall does not claim that his pollen pills are a cure for arthritis, but there is some evidence that they may bring relief to sufferers.

What happened in the case of Miss C., he believes, is that the pollen restored her vitality by providing vitamins, enzymes, microelements and amino acids. As a result her body was revitalized and could cope more ably with the problem of arthritis. Perhaps these essential food factors even stimulated the regrowth of collagen connective tissues or 'cushioning' of her spinal joints and thereby eased her back pains.

At the risk of some repetition, it must be emphasized that Pollen-B is not a medicine but a supplementary food and no medical claims are made for it; but obviously a food supplement which, in its natural state contains many good factors, often lacking as we grow older, may revitalize us and enable us to cope with illness and weaknesses.

Every individual, out of more than fifty who were originally tested with daily amounts of bee-collected pollen, reported benefits and good effects within a couple of months. These effects were pronounced and every consumer was surprised and pleased by the results so decisively achieved.

*

Mrs M. walked smartly into the first-floor coffee lounge of a local department store with the mischievous air of someone about to play a practical joke. She saw her friends and waved across the room as she approached them. She wore a gay hat but no glasses (for who needs glasses?). And it was only when she came close, swaying slightly in the elegant manner of a movie queen that you realized she was not quite as young as you had thought.

But you would never have guessed that Mrs M. was in her nineties . . . more sixty-ish perhaps. Nor would you ever guess her age from her lively, provocative way of talking. You would never guess it, either, from the smoothness of her skin or the sparkle in her eyes, and you would never realize that she had quite recently broken her leg from a fall in a supermarket. 'They pushed me,' she exclaims mischievously, 'but it was great fun in hospital with everybody waiting on me, hand and foot, and when I left they all turned out to say good-bye as if it was the queen leaving.'

Mrs M. had walked in to meet her friends – Mrs H. and Mrs W. and there was also Mr F. – they meet almost every day, these four, and talk or argue about what is going on in the world. ('Mostly we fight,' said Mrs M.)

Sometimes they are joined by Neil Lyall, who likes to know how they are all going on. For the quartet are also among his guinea-pigs, though in a rather different category. Mrs H. is over eighty, Mrs W. and Mr F. are getting on for eighty and all three have been taking Pollen-B for more than a year. They all feel that it does them good. Well, if all three survived to become centenarians it would be more than just coincidence. Lyall expects Mrs M. to reach the age of a hundred in good shape. She is a natural, he thinks, and there are comparatively few years to go.

Until recently Mrs M. still drove a car, and is proud of the fact that she has had a driving licence since she was eighteen. Her first cars were like the vintage vehicles which take part in the annual Old Crocks race to Brighton but she has had so many different cars that she has forgotten what makes most of them were.

When people ask her how she manages to look so young Mrs M. says that she has had a wonderfully happy life and still enjoys it (quite apart from the fact that she has never been short of money). But it is perhaps more than a coincidence that she used to eat a lot of home-produced honey from her own domestic hives. 'We had a dozen hives – I used to live on the stuff,' she says. And, of course, this grade of honey

131

contained a high proportion of bee-collected pollen.

It is not, however, only the middle-aged and elderly who seem to benefit from this food supplement. Among the many people Lyall selected as test subjects were several in their thirties, men and women struggling to make their way in the world, working long hours and finding themselves 'whacked' at weekends.

There was Douglas E., for example. Douglas was running a coffee lounge he owned. It was (and still is) a popular place, specializing in health foods. In addition, Douglas undertakes private catering jobs for organizations running evening parties, which often means a twelve- to fourteen-hour day. So it was hardly surprising that he was feeling whacked when Lyall introduced him to Pollen-B. Within a few weeks of taking this, he says, he found himself beginning to perk up. Work seemed less of an effort and he took the long hours in his stride. Now, he often plays squash in the evenings, and at weekends indulges in water ski-ing at Poole Harbour.

Then there was Mrs J.M. who, with her husband, runs a busy newsagent's shop. When Lyall first met her she was ill and depressed as a result of several surgical operations and, on top of it all, a motoring accident. Her husband thought she would be laid up for at least a year. But within a few weeks of taking the special pollen she was 'skipping around like a teenager' and putting in many hours a week at the shop . . . and still feeling on top of the world. She says that her relatives, living in Belfast, have found Pollen-B very beneficial. Her assistant at the shop, Mrs M. (and her husband, too), are taking bee-collected pollen with the expected good effect. And Mrs M. neither looks nor feels her age.

Since Pollen-B has become widely available in chemists

and health food stores hundreds of people have testified to feeling better for it. Not the least of these is millionaire Herman Van Vlymen, former head of the giant Scot-Bowyer group, who was thinking of retirement when he read press reports on the value of Lyall's pollen.

He wrote to Lyall:

The day I read the advertisement in the *Evening Standard* for your wonderful tablets, Pollen-B, will be a day I will not forget. Since that day my health has improved and I do not look back.

They enable me to work twelve hours a day without any ill feelings even though I am nearly seventy-three. My doctor, who makes fortnightly examinations of me, is astonished at my health. . . I recommend your Pollen-B tablets wherever I go and to all my friends and they are, without exception, taking them regularly and finding them beneficial to their health.

I wish you the very best of luck. May I also say that you have done a marvellous job for mankind.

Conclusions

After many years of painstaking research ... and the explanations in this book, it may be wise to summarize briefly the conclusions reached by Neil Lyall during his work.

First, it should be made clear that when he first realized that many people were still working at the ages of 130 years and upwards in some parts of the world he was determined to investigate and find out why these peoples lived so much longer than anyone else and also why they retained their vitality, their energy and their good health and freedom from disease.

Examination of their diets, mode of living, habits and general behaviour revealed that they all had one dietary supplement in common. While the Hunzas, for example, use crude, unstrained honey to sweeten the raw apricots which form a major item of their diet, the peoples of Azerbaydzhan scrape 'honey scrap' from the beehive floors when cleaning them. They retain and eat this, for the public, even in Azerbaydzhan, prefer the clear, sparkling honey, which is mainly sugar – while the hive scrapings contain a high proportion of bee-collected pollen like the thick, unstrained honey of South American states. The home-produced heather honey of Northern Scotland also contains a substantial amount of bee pollen and where this type of honey is eaten longevity has been noticed.

Subsequent investigations established the fact that there was nothing unusual, in these regions of longevity, for people to reach ages of 150 years and more in perfect health.

The declarations of Mankovsky and other noted gerontologists have confirmed and authenticated Neil Lyall's theories at every stage. And he took the precaution of provisionally patenting the product in several countries of the world, so that imitations or infringements would be discouraged.

A long series of meetings and consultations have been held with the authorities and it is already several years since Lyall established 'usage' of the product . . . and its name. The aid of a leading Public Analyst was enlisted and friendly relations with the leading pharmacists were established.

The main conclusions reached are based on the fact that Pollen-B appears to have similar revitalizing effects upon people living in Britain as it does upon the peoples of the Caucasus, Ecuador and Hunza who have been dependent, of course, upon beehive-scrap or thick, unstrained honey.

Neil Lyall has achieved the conversion of the active principle, namely bee-collected pollen, into a convenient, easy-to-take tablet. It is in many ways too early to know what the ultimate results will be, but, judging by the restoration of vitality in other regions of the world, it may well be a remarkable achievement.

It has been said by many leading scientists that polyvitamins, enzymes, microelements and amino acids, when administered together, can boost the health of the elderly and counteract ageing.

Bee-collected pollen is one of the very few materials which contains small but adequate amounts of all these vital food factors and, in the form of Pollen-B tablets, it can be obtained from chemists and health food stores everywhere.

Restoration of youthful vitality has been placed within the reach of everyone.

Appendix 1
Lee Foundation pollen analysis

According to the Lee Foundation analysis, bee-collected pollen contains the following enzymes:

Amylase	Diastase	Phosphatase	Lactic Dehydrogenase
Pectase	Catalase	Diaphorase	Succinic Dehydrogenase
Saccharase	Cozymase	Cytochrome Systems	(11 enzymes)

MINERALS (microelements)

Calcium	Phosphorus	Iron	Copper
Potassium	Magnesium	Sodium	Manganese
Sulphur	Titanium	Silicon	(11 minerals)

*

It should be noted that the bees, when gathering pollen, during the collection of nectar for honey-making, add a little nectar and saliva in order to make it adhere more firmly to their legs. It is not known what factors may be added to the pollen but it seems certain that it contains hormones, which can be beneficial in trace quantities.

The other main ingredients of pollen include polyvitamins and amino acids as follows:

VITAMINS

Provitamin A (Carotenoids)	Vitamin K
Vitamin D	Vitamin E
Vitamin B1 (Thiamine or Aneurine)	Biotin
Choline	Folic acid
Inositol	Vitamin B6 (pyridoxine)
Vitamin B12 (cyanocobalamin)	Rutin
Pantothenic acid	(14 vitamins)
Vitamin C (Ascorbic acid)	

The synergistic effect of a wide range of vitamins is far more important than a larger quantity of one or two isolated vitamins and the polyvitamins recommended to boost the health of the elderly are sufficient to rectify any marginal deficiency.

AMINO ACIDS (constituents of proteins)

Tryptophane	Lysine	Methionine	Threonine
Phenylalanine	Valine	Isoleucine	Leucine
Cystine	Arginine	Histidine	Tyrosine
Glutamic acid	Serine	Proline	Hydroxyproline
Glycine	Alanine	Aspartic acid	(19 amino acids)

These amino acids are the building materials of the human body; and stimulants or catalysts are, of course, useless without the building materials for cells and tissues. Since bee-collected pollen contains an average of 20 per cent amino acids, this is likely to be sufficient to rectify any deficiency and enable body processes to function normally. The major fatty acids present in pollens are Oleic and Stearic. Linoleic, Palmitic, Caproic and about ten other fatty acids are present in trace amounts. Pollen also contains Lecithin, Nuclein,

140

Guanine and other ingredients, again in trace quantities.

There are several ingredients which are known to be non-deleterious but which have not yet been identified. Hormones are known to be components of bee-collected pollen and these probably include traces of insulin and thyroxine.

Other factors include an antibiotic factor, a growth factor and, according to Wm Robinson, USA Dept of Agriculture, an anticarcinogenic factor.

It seems likely, therefore, that when more work has been carried out on the components of pollen, further benefits from the consumption of this material may be revealed.

Appendix 2
Other scientists' opinions

One of the most informative papers on the chemical composition and nutritional value of pollens collected by bees was a result of the work of Vivino and Palmer at the University of Minnesota, USA. But many British scientists are now interested in the potential value of pollen in medical fields.

At the present stage it is only possible to regard pollen as a natural food supplement. When a great deal more work has been done on investigating the ingredients of pollens it may be that many results of benefit to mankind will follow. Scientists at the Ministry of Agriculture, Fisheries and Food have already recognized the value of pollens as supplementary foods and so has the Department of Health. Medical specialists have expressed surprise at the effects of consuming bee-collected pollen. But there the matter rests until more research is undertaken.

Researches are already being carried out in France, America, Germany and other countries. Palynology is a relatively new science. Clinical trials and innumerable tests must be completed before the whole story can be revealed. But Nicolai Tsitsin and Neil Lyall have already linked the eating of bee-collected pollen with long, healthy lives and freedom from many ailments which afflict mankind. It appears that Pollen-B, for example, enables athletes to give peak performances and acquire more energy and vitality. Performances at the 1974 Commonwealth Games, by athletes trained on Pollen-B, seem to bear witness to this very satisfactory result.

Appendix 3
Testimony from users of Pollen-B

This is a sample of hundreds of unsolicited letters received from people who take pollen tablets regularly.

'...It is now over nine months since I first started your course of Pollen-B. The benefits are really too numerous to recount ...suffice it to say that, at the age of sixty-four I have regained the energy of when I was forty...
Mr W., Hazel Grove, Cheshire

'...I have been taking one tablet of Pollen-B each day for the past six months ... as an OAP I find Pollen-B enables me to continue in full employment out-of-doors as a gardener in all weathers ... Those rheumatic pains seem to have vanished ... Pollen-B certainly is most helpful to keep me feeling fit and healthy...'
Mr A.T., Sussex

'... My husband is ill ... he had an accident and all his hair came off but after taking two packs of Pollen-B it is coming back and he says he feels much better himself.'
Mrs H., Sheffield

'... As a diabetic of many years ... having witnessed the amazing effect of this product on my family I admit taking it for one week only and I still cannot realize that in that short period I walked with a skip in step that made me think I was twenty years younger and I frightened myself with the speed I was able to do my household tasks...'
Mrs B., Halesowen, Worcs

'... I am seventy-five and my wife is sixty-nine and after taking Pollen-B for just a fortnight we found a great improvement in health and wellbeing ... I was more mentally alert and physically vigorous than I have ever been for the last twenty years and my hair which was pure white, is now changing colour...'
Mr A.T., Manchester

'... While I have been taking Pollen-B I have never felt better ... always having suffered stomach upsets and lack of appetite ... I can eat a full meal and feel no uneasiness at all after it. I cannot praise them highly enough...'
Mr C.P., Barton-on-Humber

'... I've been on Pollen-B for some time now and find them excellent. I'm sixty-eight years old and have more energy and less aches and pains than for years...'
Mr M., Clacton-on-Sea, Essex

'... I started taking Pollen-B tablets last July. Since then they have had a marked effect on my health. For years I have suffered from migraine headaches; have tried every known form of medication including visits to a migraine clinic; up to taking Pollen-B nothing worked. If anything, the headaches were becoming more chronic.

However, in the past nine months I have suffered less and less and I know that this is on account of the Pollen-B tablets. Coupled with this I am less tense and this has had unexpected effects such as not being dependent on laxatives, which I had taken regularly for years . . . It's marvellous after years of suffering to be free of the pain of bad migraines, also the necessity of constantly taking analgesics . . .'
Mr J.E.K., Stroud, Glos

'. . . I underwent a serious operation and my recovery has been long and painful . . . I began to take Pollen-B tablets [about six months ago]. I am now fully recovered and feel remarkably well . . . in my opinion the tablets have contributed in no small measure to this end . . .'
Mr H.S., Isle of Man

Appendix 4
Athletes and sportsmen

While there is testimony that Pollen-B is a boon to the elderly, it has become a popular energy-booster and stamina-builder among British athletes and sportsmen. For some time, national coach Tom McNab has been an enthusiastic consumer of bee-collected pollen.

Many of the peak performances achieved at the Commonwealth Games in 1974 are thought to be due to the widespread consumption of Pollen-B by competitors. No less than thirteen gold medals and twelve silver medals were won by British athletes.

In February 1974, the *Observer* published the fact that Judy Vernon, the unexpected hurdles champion, had admitted feeling 'generally more energetic' but was even more impressed by the fact that she 'hadn't had a cold since taking pollen'.

The *Sunday Times*, in May 1974, confirmed that Geoff Capes the sensational shot-putter had been consuming bee-collected pollen, too, and other athletes who have improved their performances include David Jenkins, Colin O'Neill and Donna Murray. David Jenkins has said that he is 'very happy with Pollen-B'.

The results obtained by taking bee-collected pollen seem to

have aroused the interest of young and old alike. But especially in the field of sport. Coaches and players are becoming more and more interested.

Appendix 5
Future medical applications

The Institut Jules Bordet in Brussels, which is involved with the National Cancer Institute in America, has undertaken to test and evaluate Lyall's stabilized pollen in cancer research.

Another surprising effect of Pollen-B tablets is their apparent easing of arthritic pains. Several instances of this have been reported.

While Neil Lyall is primarily concerned with food science and the beneficial effects of dietary supplements, it seems that medical interest in at least three aspects of potential benefits in so-called 'incurable diseases' must at least be encouraged and every assistance given. The fact that Lyall's bee-collected pollen may be useful in combating serious afflictions – although many further tests have yet to be made – is at least an indication of the potential usefulness of the product in the relief of suffering.

It may, of course, take a year or two for tests to be completed but one must welcome the initial medical interest. The primitive agrarian peoples who have – possibly by sheer accident – helped to reveal the beneficial effects of this food supplement may never have imagined that this simple product of remote regions could have such potentially wide applications.

Within the next few years it seems possible that additional

uses and applications will be found for bee-collected pollen. When the prophet Mahomet described a product of the bees as 'containing the healing of mankind' he may not have been exaggerating the future scope of this grade of pollen.

As a prophylactic for the prevention of the common cold it seems that yet another opportunity exists for this application. It has already been brought to Lyall's attention that consumers of Pollen-B have not had a cold since taking it. This is not by any means a claim but a report on the fact that it seems to protect the epithelial tissues from airborne infections like the common cold, influenza and so on. On questioning many users of Pollen-B, Lyall has been pleasantly surprised to learn that consumers have mostly reported being 'free from colds'. And this again was unexpected.

Appendix 6 Life expectancy at birth in Great Britain

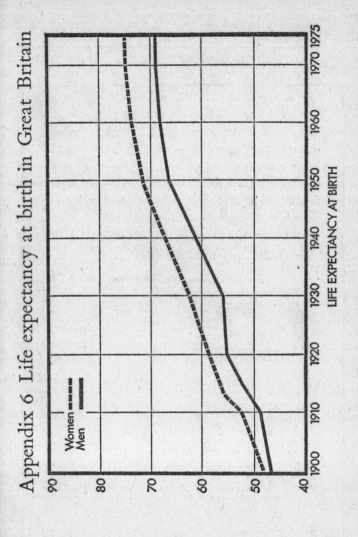

LIFE EXPECTANCY AT BIRTH

Appendix 7
Areas of Longevity

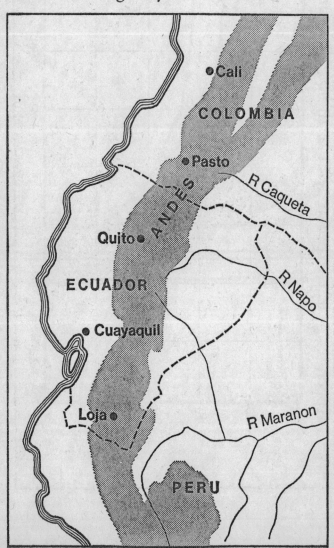

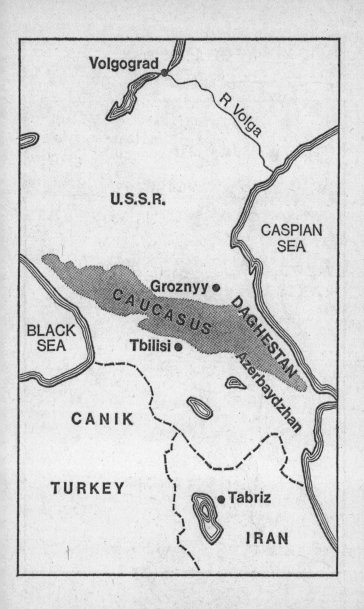

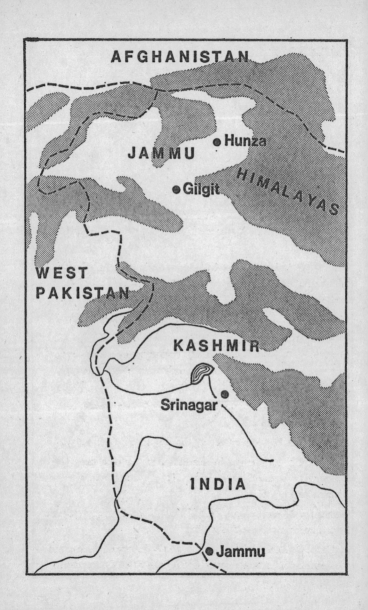

Appendix 8
Bibliography and references

Auclair, J. L. and Jamieson, C. A. 'Qualitative Analysis of amino acids in pollen collected by bees', *Science* 108 (1948) 137

Chauvin, R. 'Chemical Composition and Biological Value of Pollen' (mimeograph) Apicultural Research Station, Bures-sur-Yvette, France

Chauvin, R. and others, 'A substance occurring in pollen which inhibits the development of certain bacteria', *A.R.Sci. (Sci.) Biol. Paris* 146 (1952) 645

Comfort, Alex *Ageing – The Biology of Senescence*, Routledge & Kegan Paul (1964)

Dutcher, R. A. 'Vitamin Studies III, Observation on the curative properties of honey, nectar and corn pollen in avian polyneuritis', *Journal of Biological Chemistry* 36 (1918) 551

Erdtman, G. 'Literature on Palynology', *Geol. Foren. Stockh. Forh.* 72; *Chemical Abstracts* 44 (1950) 6786e

Hillemann, H. H. Modern Nutrition (16) 3 21–27 (March 1963)

Ichikawa, Ch. 'Biochemical Studies of Pollen', *Journal of the Agricultural Chemical Society of Japan* 12 (1936) 1117; *Chemical Abstracts* 31 (1937) 2640

Lenhoff, H. M. and Loomis, W. F. *Time, Cells and Ageing*, Academic Press, London and New York (1962)

McCance, R. A. and Widdowson, A. M. 'A Fantasy on Ageing and the Bearing of Nutrition upon it' CIBA Foundation Colloquia on Ageing 1 (1955) 186

McCay, C. M. and Crowell, M. F. 'Prolonging the Life-Span', *Scientific Monthly* 39 (1934) 405

Okonuki, K. 'Coenzymes in Pollen', *Science* (Japan) 12 (1942) 221; *Chemical Abstracts* 45 (1951) 10309a

Robinson, W. 'Delay in the Appearance of Palpable Mammary Tumors in Mice Following the Ingestion of Pollenized Food', *Journal of the National Cancer Institute* 9 (1948) 119

Sherman, H. C. and Campbell, H. L. 'Rate of growth and Length of Life', *Proceedings of the National Academy of Science* 21, 235

Shock, N. W. 'Metabolism in Old Age', *Geriatrics* 232

Silberberg, M. and Silberberg, R. 'Diet and Life-Span', *Physiological Review* 35 (1951) 347–62

Szilard, L. 'On the Nature of the Ageing Process', *Proceedings of the National Academy of Science* 45, 30–45

Thoms, W. J. *The Longevity of Man: its facts and fictions*, London (1873)

'Vitamin Content of Bee Foods', *Journal of Economic Entomology* 33 (1940) 396

Vivino, A. E. and Palmer, L. S. 'The Chemical Composition and Nutritional Value of Pollens Collected by Bees', *Archives of Biochemistry and Biophysics* 4 (1944) 129

Yacob, M. and Swaroop, S. 'Longevity and Old Age in the Punjab', *British Medical Journal* 2 (1945) 433

Yakushkina, N. I. 'The Growth Substance in Pollen', *Doklady Akad Nauk SSSR*, 56 (1947) 549; *Chemical Abstracts* 43 (1949) 7553d

Young, T. E. *On Centenarians and the Duration of the Human Race* London, Layton (1899)

Glossary

AGEING A slowing down of body metabolism and tempo, often due to the natural tendency of the elderly to eat an 'unbalanced diet' of tea and biscuits, buttered toast and jam and not enough meat, fruit and vegetables. This self-conditioning can, of course, cause deficiency diseases. These can be prevented indefinitely by taking a dietary supplement of the missing essential food factors

AMINO ACIDS Constituents of proteins which in turn compose a large part of all living matter

ANAEMIA Lack of red blood corpuscles – which carry oxygen round the body. Can be remedied by eating liver and taking soluble iron salts in tablet form combined with Vitamin B12 (Cyanocobalamin)

ARTERIO-SCLEROSIS Hardening of the arteries

ARTHRITIS Inflammation of the joints caused by breakdown of the collagen connective tissue or 'cushioning'

CELLS The units of protoplasm, containing a nucleus and cytoplasm. All tissue is made up of individual cells. The average cell is so small it can only be seen under a microscope

CHOLESTEROL A waxy substance in the tissues of the body. Performs useful functions but excess is very harmful, causing furring and clogging up of the arteries with resultant heart troubles

DIABETES A disease causing excessive glucose (sugar) in the blood and urine. Sometimes caused by failure of the pancreas to produce insulin

ENZYMES Organic catalysts or stimulants essential to body metabolism. Each enzyme is specific to its own particular type of stimulation . . . Enzymes are vital to the proper utilization of food

GERIATRICS The treatment of the aged

GERONTOLOGY The study of ageing and the aged

HAEMOGLOBIN Red colouring pigment of the blood. Is able to carry oxygen to various parts of the body in the form of oxyhaemoglobin; also to combine with oxygen in the lungs

HORMONE A substance produced by an endocrine gland in the body, and regulating functions of the organism

MICROELEMENTS Inorganic elements which have mineral salts essential to the correct functioning of the body . . . like calcium, potassium and iron salts which are essential food factors

PALYNOLOGY The study of pollen and its components

PROTEINS Organic compounds which comprise a large part of all living matter. These are vital in our food and are built into the body tissues

SENESCENCE Growing old, or the period of advanced age

SENILE Manifesting the behaviour typical of old age

TUMOUR (Malignant) Local swelling due to morbid growth of cells and tending to recur after removal by surgery. An intake of bee-collected pollen is reported to have retarded tumours in mice and rats

VITAMINS Accessory food factors essential in normal diets. Their absence can lead to deficiency diseases. Deficiency of vitamin A for example can cause night-blindness. Deficiency of vitamin C can cause Scurvy